Permanent Results

without

Permanent Dieting

the

D0062523

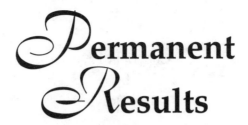

Curves®

WEIGHT-LOSS METHOD

Written by
Health & Nutrition Counselor
Gary Heavin
Founder & C.E.O., Curves International Inc.
The World's Largest Fitness Center Franchise

Copyright 1999
by
Gary Heavin

5th Edition — 2002

Edited By Linda Heavin-Britton
Illustrations By Virginia Heavin

Published by
Curves Intl., Inc.
400 Schroeder
Waco, TX 76710

Printed in U.S.A.

Dedication

As a very young man, someone taught me the power of positive thinking. He showed me how to be solution concious rather than problem concious. I learned from him the value of setting goals and that obstacles are a part of the experience that make the journey worthwhile. He showed me that a "big shot" is just a little shot that keeps on shooting. He convinced me that I could achieve whatever my mind could perceive. He was and is the best teacher one could have because he taught by example. Whatever I know about persistence, commitment, and the courage to stand for what I believe, I owe to my older brother, David Heavin. I dedicate this book to him.

THE CURVES STORY

As the founder and C.E.O. of the world's largest fitness center franchise, Curves International, Inc., it is my privilege to share the most innovative discoveries of exercise and weight control. Over twenty-seven years ago, I opened my first women's fitness facility and began to coach and guide women through the process of attaining optimal health and weight.

Through the years I developed or made available the most effective methods of health and weight management. They include:

*A strength-training program for women

*Thirty-minute total fitness for busy schedules

*Quality fitness centers designed for women

*Exercise and nutritional guidance in the same location

*A temporary dieting method that produces permanent results

We currently have almost four thousand Curves locations in fifty states and six nations. On average, we open a new location every four hours.

I wish I could say that I figured this out easily and recently. I was a pre-med major in college twenty-seven years ago. I was learning about physiology at the cellular level. I was not exposed to the standard nutritional information but rather how the human body functions. In other words, I learned how to learn about exercise and weight-loss, but I had no bias. I was free to seek the truth.

At age twenty, I had been working to put myself through college, and it was becoming apparent that I couldn't afford medical school. An opportunity arose whereby I could take over a fitness center in Houston, Texas. The facility was about to go out of business when I stepped in. I knew nothing about running a fitness center but I knew about caring for people. I realized that this was an opportunity to treat people before they became ill.

I began to take responsibility for the results that the members expected. As their personal trainer, I would teach them the proper method to lift weights and combine cardio training. I would weigh and measure them monthly, have them keep food diaries and advise them on their diets. Soon I began to hold weight-loss seminars and six-week challenges with the members. At weekly meetings, I would monitor calorie intakes and results as well as discuss willpower and support.

I was successful enough to acquire a second location in just over a year. Within a few years, I owned six "women only" fitness centers. I was soon counseling with hundreds of women through weekly weight-loss seminars. By the time I was thirty I owned fourteen centers with fifty-thousand members. I had written *The Sweet Joy of Sugar Free Living*, which utilized the higher-protein, lower-carbohydrate approach to dieting and the Heavin formula for metabolic change.

In my early thirties, I suffered financially through the learning process of experience. However, I retained the information of many years of coaching and counseling and believed that I could create the most effective health and weight-loss methods for women.

My wife, Diane, and I opened the first Curves in Harlingen, Texas in August of 1992. We were immediately successful but patiently waited until two years later to open the second location.

With hundreds of members acquiring the habit of exercise and successfully losing weight, we realized that we should share this program. Franchising seemed to be the perfect vehicle. This concept was best offered by a local person with a passion for helping other people. In October of 1995, we opened the first Curves franchise in Paris, Texas. Within ninety days we sold ten franchises. By the end of the first year we had fifty locations. At the end of the second year we had two hundred and fifty locations. By the end of the third year we had almost six hundred franchises and today we are well on our way to many thousands of locations.

Curves has received many accolades over the last few years. *Entrepreneur* magazine has chosen Curves for the following awards: Number 1 Best New Franchise (two years in a row), Number 3 Best of All Franchises (last year), and Third Fastest Growing Franchise (last year). After just seven years in business, we now have one Curves for every three McDonald's locations in America. This is a testament to the effectiveness of our program.

I recently took the time to complete my formal degree in Health and Nutrition Counseling. Curves is currently underwriting research at Baylor University in an effort to scientifically validate our theories in a laboratory environment. Over one million women are acquiring the habit of exercise and moving away from obesity and chronic disease with the help of our program.

The secret to our success is quite simple. Thirty-minute fitness is something women find the time to do. A total workout is essential to lasting results, especially strength training. A convenient, comfortable environment is motivating. Quality nutritional guidance in the same place that you exercise is important. A temporary method of dieting with the ability to raise metabolism will enable permanent results without permanent dieting.

There is another aspect that has assured Curves' success. This company has been established on the solid biblical principles of integrity, unity and service. God's will is sought in our business decisions, and then we do our best to carry it out. This commitment includes treating people honestly and fairly and has allowed us to build relationships rather than to just sell franchises or memberships. The astounding growth of this company is His signature. He has provided the opportunity to serve.

I write this book to help you escape from the bondage of poor health and obesity. Curves' innovations have helped thousands of women achieve success with their health and weight-loss goals. The Curves' program requires your effort. It may be the toughest part of your day, but it works. Allow me to share the Curves' mission statement:

> "We commit our methods and motivation
> to help people to help themselves in their quest
> to attain a better quality of life."

If you have any health concerns, you should see a physician before beginning this or any other fitness and weight-loss program.

CHAPTER I

THE PHYSIOLOGY OF FITNESS

The Price of Good Health Is a Bargain

Have you been paying the price for not exercising? If you are overweight, how many hours a day do you spend thinking about your weight? Most women tell me every waking moment, and some even dream about it. Feeling bad about yourself usually affects your marriage, parenting, job, even your spiritual life. Then there are the health costs of preventable illnesses and probably less years and certainly less quality years of your life. Are you sick and tired of being sick and tired?

What's the price for controlling your weight and protecting your health? With Curves it's thirty minutes a few times each week. The price also includes eating healthy foods and taking a good vitamin and mineral supplement, and some of you might need to temporarily diet to lose any excess body fat. Doesn't it sound like the cost for good health is a bargain compared to the price of not exercising? It's really an easy decision. You can exchange all of the hours and misery of not taking care of yourself for thirty minutes three times a week. In fact, you will enjoy the small cost of good health.

There Ain't No Free Lunch
But There Is a Blue-Plate Special

Have you ever seen those tables that you lay on that are supposed to shake the fat off of you? They often come with tanning facilities. I call them "shake and bakes." Do you believe that laying on a moving table can burn excess fat from your body while you just lay there? When it comes to most things, you don't get something for nothing.

Progress has created the technology that allows us to escape from most physical labor. **The price of this progress is either illness or exercise.**

Efficient Fitness — Burn Calories Not Time

You can, however, efficiently exercise. I believe that the Curves workout is the most efficient method of complete exercise. It changes your shape faster than any other activity. In just thirty minutes you perform all five of the components of exercise.

1. Warm up
2. Twenty minutes of sustained target heart rate (cardio)
3. Three sets of strength training on all major muscle groups
4. Cool down
5. Stretching (elasticity)

Total Fitness Is Essential

Each of these components is necessary for optimal health and weight-loss. When you can accomplish them all in just 30 minutes, it becomes "medicine that you'll take." When it is safe, pleasant, and fun, it becomes a habit that you will acquire. Most women who join Curves have never before been able to stick with an exercise program. Here, they find the environment comfortable, and they enjoy visiting with their friends. In as little as a few weeks, they have energy, their clothes are fitting looser, and they feel better about themselves.

The Curves breakthrough is "hydraulic resistance." Strength training machines alternate with aerobic recovery stations. You change stations every 30 seconds as you move around the circuit three times. Heart rates are checked every eight minutes to allow you to adjust your intensity to stay at your target level. Hydraulic resistance is safe like aquatic exercise yet better in that you are able to isolate muscle groups and create adequate resistance to overload the muscle. The first and the last few minutes are slowly performed for warm up and cool down. You end your 30-minute workout with a stretching routine.

Successful Losers Exercise

How important is exercise to permanent weight-loss? The National Weight Control Registry, maintained by the University of Pittsburgh School of Medicine and the University of Colorado School of Health Sciences, is the largest ongoing observation program. They track people who have lost thirty or more pounds and have kept it off for at least a year. They found that 94% of successful losers increased their physical activity and 92% are continuing to exercise to maintain their weight-loss.[1]

Curves members have enjoyed a window of opportunity. Almost four out of five reach their body-fat goals without having to diet. If they have twenty pounds or less to lose and give up sugar, most of them reach their goals with exercise alone.

This phenomenon occurs because our average new member has never regularly exercised and her metabolism is high due to the sugar that she, like most others, is eating. When she begins to burn several hundred calories per workout, strength train, and quit eating sugar, her body will quickly respond.

The Missing Link ... Strength Training

The big news in exercise is strength training. Many of you have been unable to reach your body fat goals or keep your weight off by doing traditional aerobics, walking, stair climbing, swimming, or jumping to conclusions. These can be an important part of your exercise program, but you are missing a major component.

Dr. Wayne Westcott, a researcher for Y.M.C.A.s of America, reported the following study. Over an eight-week period, one group of aerobic exercisers performed thirty minutes of aerobics three times per week. The second group performed fifteen minutes of strength training and fifteen minutes of aerobics three times per week. The aerobic-only group lost three pounds of body fat but also lost a half pound of muscle. The strength trainers lost ten pounds of body fat and gained a pound and a half of muscle.[2]

	Body-fat	Muscle
Aerobics only	-3 lbs	-1/2 lbs
Aerobics & Strength training	-10 lbs	+1 1/2 lbs

Would you like to lose body fat three times faster? Would you like to keep it off? Then you've got to strength train.

Muscles Burn Calories

Muscles are the engines of our bodies. A pound of muscle burns about fifty calories per day at rest. **When you walk, do aerobics, or just diet to lose weight, up to forty percent of your weight-loss is lean tissue or muscle.** If you have lost twenty pounds on a diet, up to eight pounds may be muscle. That means that you have lowered your metabolism by as much as four hundred calories per day. Is it any wonder that you gained your weight back and then some?

True strength training requires that you "overload the muscle." You must move a greater resistance than the muscle is accustomed to. This progressive increase in resistance stimulates the muscle to increase in size and strength. Larger and more activated muscle fibers result in a higher metabolism.

Resistance Training Resists Muscle Loss

The human body adapts to behavior. Your body prioritizes muscles when you are using them in a strength training activity. It protects muscles from tissue loss. You can lose only body fat while burning stored energy. In other words, you can lose twenty pounds without losing eight pounds of muscle. You will even gain a few pounds of muscle. For the first time in your life, you can have the hope of permanent results without permanent dieting. **For the first time, your metabolism will be higher after losing weight than when you began to lose weight.**

Chuck Steak to Sirloin

Just a few years ago, I had to assure women that they would not look like Arnold Swarzenegger if they strength trained. Most women are now aware that they will not get big, bulky muscles without tremendous effort. Have you ever seen a pound of chuck steak next to a pound of sirloin in the meat case? They weigh the same but the chuck steak is larger because fat is less dense than lean tissue. When you start with a high percentage of body fat, you will have part of that fat throughout the muscle. Your muscles will be like chuck steak. As you burn stored fat, you will also burn some from the muscles. You will turn your muscles from chuck to sirloin. You'll end up with firm, strong muscles but not necessarily larger looking muscles. Your muscles will weigh more, but they will use far more energy.

Use It to Not Lose It

According to Dr. Jack Wilmore at the University of Texas, "We know that resting metabolic rate goes down 3% per decade, and the limited research we have suggests that's mostly due to the loss of muscle mass."[3] In a study conducted at Pennsylvania State University using the Curves workout with a group of seniors averaging seventy-five years of age, we found that they acquired significant gains in muscle size and strength during a nine-week program.[4] This ability to restore muscle and metabolism is great news in the Battle of the Bulge—your bulge.

There are many other benefits with resistance training. Your muscles provide greater stability to help prevent you from falling or injuring yourself if you do fall. Many older people break their hips and do not recover due to a lack of muscle. Strong muscles provide joint support and are critical to healing most back problems.

Safe-Fast-Effective-Fitness

The Curves workout allows you to perform three sets of

strength training exercises for all major muscle groups while you sustain your target heart rate. It is not only time efficient, but the resistance is safer. You are pulling and pushing, rather than lifting and lowering. Eighty-five percent of injuries that occur in a gym happen during the lowering of the weight. This lowering of the weight is the "eccentric" contraction. The Curves workout eliminates the eccentric contraction with its double-positive movement. This also eliminates almost all soreness. Opposing muscle groups are worked symmetrically (on both sides) for a balanced workout. In addition, you are working two muscle groups at the same time. This allows you to perform three sets on all major muscle groups, completed in just thirty minutes.

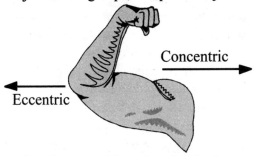

Concentric

Eccentric

Another feature with hydraulics is that resistance is determined by speed. The faster you go the harder it is. With weight stack or free weight training, you are moving a fixed weight. As you go through the range of motion, leverage and momentum cause the weight to become easy, and you do not overload the muscle for most of the range of motion. With our program, as you move faster, the resistance is harder. This results in overloading the muscle the full range of motion. The muscle will firm its full length. This creates a better look as well as provides the best method of increasing power. Power is the functional aspect of strength. Power allows you to lift your child, get out of bed, or hit a tennis ball.

When you first see the Curves workout system, don't be fooled by the lack of weight stacks. You are about to experience the toughest thirty minutes of your day. Yet, you'll find that it is fast, fun, and effective. It will help you to acquire the habit of exercise.

Aerobic Exercise for the Health of It

Aerobic exercise is defined as an activity that allows the muscles to utilize oxygen in their energy processes. During a short burst of effort, such as sprinting, muscles will burn primarily glycogen or glucose. **If you perform an activity that raises your heart rate to a training or "target" level and sustain that rate for more than ten minutes or so, you are working aerobically.**

As the heart is a muscle, it must be strengthened by progressively increasing its work load. A stronger heart will pump more blood with each beat. As the entire cardio-respiratory system is exercised, your lungs more efficiently process oxygen and impurities. Your vascular system responds more appropriately and blood pressure often lowers. Your muscles are able to utilize energy better and rid themselves of waste. The more and the larger muscle groups that are involved in your workout, the quicker your body begins to benefit from exercise. By working all the major muscle groups during your workout, your cardiovascular-respiratory system more quickly responds.

Pace Yourself

Heart rate is a simple method of determining your workout intensity. It is important that you work hard enough to strengthen your heart. It is also important that you not work too hard and put yourself at risk. You can check your heart rate easily by counting your carotid or radial (wrist) pulse. Your target heart rate for aerobic exercise should be between fifty and eighty percent of your maximum heart rate. A simple formula for target heart rate is:

220 - AGE = MAXIMUM HEART RATE
X 50% TO 80% = TARGET HEART RATE

Example for a fifty year old in good health:

220 - 50 = 170 (Maximum Heart Rate)

X 65% = 110 (Target Heart Rate)

If you are just beginning an exercise program or if you have any of the following conditions, 50% of maximum heart rate would be an appropriate beginning target. Any of these conditions might require seeking the advice of your doctor before you begin:

Obesity   Diabetes   Heart Problems

High Blood Pressure   Pregnancy

Back Problems

With the Curves workout, we utilize ten-second heart rate counts. You can simply look at your age on the wall chart and see which column represents the number of beats for your percentage target. You can multiply the ten-second count by six and find your beats per minute.

Perceived Exertion

Heart rate can sometimes be ineffective as a measure of exertion for many people. If you are taking blood pressure medication, for example, you should utilize perceived exertion. Generally, if you are breathing deeply but are able to maintain a conversation during exercise, you are working at an appropriate level of intensity. If you are gasping for air and cannot speak more than a few words at a time, you're working too hard.

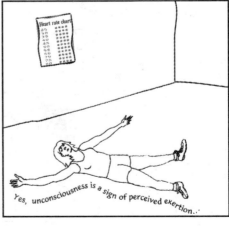

Yes, unconsciousness is a sign of perceived exertion..

Burn Fat Not Sugar

Aerobic exercise is considered essential for burning stored fat. A steady level of activity will require a steady supply of energy. Your body's gas tank is stored fat. During the first few minutes of activity, your muscles will burn primarily glucose or glycogen as energy. With the appropriate intensity, they will begin to burn more fat as the activity prolongs. As the signal is sent to fat stores that more energy is needed, the fat stores begin to give up fat to be used as energy. The fat stores don't like it, but they have no choice. The more conditioned you are, the faster your body is able to access fat as energy.

If you have not been exercising, your muscles are used to burning primarily glycogen or glucose for quick energy. For fast, limited efforts, glucose or glycogen is available in adequate amounts. Your muscles are not adapted to quickly access the fat that is available for energy. There are fat-burning enzymes that develop as you sustain activity for longer periods of time. **As you get more fit, your body will more quickly and easily be able to access fat for energy.**

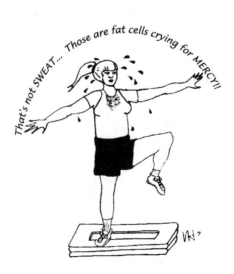

18

The key to aerobic exercise is FIT.

F is for frequency. You need to perform aerobic exercise at least three days a week to see improvement.

I is for intensity. You need to exercise at your target heart rate.

T is for time. You need to sustain your target heart rate for at least twenty minutes.

The Curves workout allows you to aerobically exercise as you perform strength-training activities. This is the best of both worlds, in half the time. Your body burns stored fat as energy while it protects and increases lean tissue and metabolism.

Warm Up and Cool Down for Safety

Warming up is best done by doing the activity you're about to do, but doing it slowly. Warming up before a workout provides numerous benefits.

Warming up...

Increases blood flow to the muscles

Allows oxygen quicker access to muscles

Speeds up the breakdown of glucose and fatty acids

Makes muscles more elastic and less susceptible to injury

Reduces heart irregularities associated with sudden exercise

More easily burns fat

With the Curves workout, the first few minutes are performed at a slow rate and then gradually increased.

Cool down is also important. The last few minutes of your workout should be done at a progressively slower rate. If your target heart rate is 120 BPM, you should be below 80 BPM upon finishing your workout. Cool down allows your body to gradually adjust back to normal.

Stretching Is Worth the Time

Stretching for elasticity is the final step in a total workout. Studies show that due to a higher body temperature, the best time to stretch is after a workout. A static stretch is a low intensity, long-duration stretch and is considered the safest method of stretching. Stretch one joint at a time. Isolate the joint and slowly elongate the muscles associated with the joint through the full range of motion. Hold the position for ten seconds and then extend a bit further. Be careful not to bounce or bob. Curves utilizes a wall poster with each of the specific stretches. You should spend a few minutes stretching following each workout.

Some of the benefits of stretching are:
* **Decreased risk of injury and enhanced joint integrity**
* **Increased blood supply and nutrients to joint structures**
* **Better balance, coordination, and situational awareness**
* **Decreased risk of lower back pain**

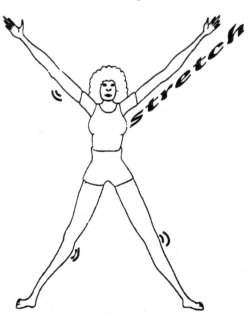

Marge loves to stretch

20

Chapter Review

*Optimal health and weight control are dependent on each of the five areas of a total workout.

*If you are strength training, you will protect and increase lean tissue, which raises metabolism.

*Aerobic exercise allows you to burn body fat and to improve your heart, lungs, and vascular system.

*Warming up and cooling down allows your body to safely adjust to the stress of exercise.

*Stretching enhances the quality of movement and the integrity of joints.

*Many women have walked or done aerobic exercise classes but have not been able to reach their weight-loss goals. Resistance training protects muscle and increases metabolism while losing body fat. With the Curves workout program, you can expect lasting results.

Curves®

CHAPTER II

UNDERSTANDING WEIGHT GAIN

- You Don't Have to Diet Forever

- Things Aren't As Bad As They Seem

- A Half-Pound of Prevention Is Worth 30 Pounds of Cure

- Postpartum Pounds

- Missed Opportunities

- Protect Us from Ourselves

- That Dreaded Evil Plateau

- Minimum of Food — Minimum of Options

- Dieting Begets Dieting

- Chapter Review

You Don't Have to Diet Forever

Conventional dieting information is primarily flawed because it requires a "life sentence" approach to weight-loss. Almost all programs approach dieting as something you must do forever. Consumer Reports rates a diet by, "Can this diet satisfy your nutritional needs indefinitely?"[5]

Weight Watchers® calls it their "maintenance program." Jenny Craig®, Nutrisystem®, and Diet Center® have variations referred to as behavior modification or other terms which simply translate: dieting forever. Even some of my favorite programs, such as Protein Power and Dr. Atkins, teach that you've got to follow their programs permanently, with only a few days off, here and there.

You might begin these programs because you are desperate, but can you really diet forever as they require? If you cannot, then you shouldn't be surprised that you failed in the past. Nor should you feel defeated by your past failures. A permanent diet embraces failure.

Things Aren't As Bad As They Seem

Let's take a look at the two most common ways that people gain weight. **First, almost everyone gains his or her weight gradually**. According to the American Research Council, the average American gains three pounds a year. Over half of all adult Americans are considered overweight. So, let's say that the overweight half are gaining all of those six pounds a year. That averages just a half-a-pound per month for each person.

With all of our poor eating and exercise habits, we, on average, are gaining only half-a-pound a month. Now that can add up. In five years, you can find yourself thirty pounds overweight, which is where most people find themselves.

A Half-Pound of Prevention Is Worth Thirty Pounds of Cure

Let me ask you this. When you put your mind to it, how

24

long does it take you to lose a half a pound? Can you do it in two or three days? A half-pound of body fat is equal to seventeen-hundred and fifty calories.

In theory, if you ate fifteen hundred calories for three days, instead of twenty-two hundred, you should have accomplished this. So isn't it reasonable to assume that if you had not changed any of your exercise or eating habits but dieted two or three days each month, that you would not have gained those thirty pounds? The answer is a resounding yes!

Can you diet two or three days a month if you don't have to diet the other twenty-nine days? Sure you can. It's time to get excited about losing weight.

Postpartum Pounds

The second way women gain weight is through an extreme body change such as pregnancy. During pregnancy, hormonal changes occur which allow the body to operate more efficiently and to more easily store excess energy as body fat. The purpose of this is to provide nutrition, insulation, and protection for the baby.

Pregnancy is an excellent example of the hormonal influences on metabolism. Can body chemistry change human metabolism and influence the sum of calories consumed with regards to body weight? Just ask a woman who has had three months of morning sickness, not eaten very well, and has gained twenty pounds during a pregnancy.

Many women have kept an extra ten pounds with each of several pregnancies. Otherwise, their weight gains have occurred slowly, like most other people.

Missed Opportunities

Breast feeding was an opportunity to lose those extra pounds. During the last twenty years, many women have had to go back to work or it just wasn't in vogue, so they didn't breast feed. They ended up with the extra weight.

Protect Us from Ourselves

We don't give the human body proper credit for its own capabilities. It protects us from becoming too obese. Look at the activity level and the eating habits of most Americans. Most of us should be hundreds of pounds overweight. Very few people are more than a hundred pounds overweight. Experts claim that the extra weight requires more muscle and energy to move, and the increase in metabolism keeps us from weighing more. You've seen a few people, on television, that weigh more than six hundred pounds. Lying there unable to move, someone brings thousands of calories to their bedside. They are not burning much energy, and their calorie intake is extraordinary. The math says, six thousand calories consumed, minus several thousand calories burned, adds almost a pound of fat every day. That's three hundred and fifty-six pounds a year, which seldom happens. My point is that there are chemical influences that affect body weight beyond exercise and calories.

That Dreaded Evil Plateau

Another perspective, with which you are more familiar, is the body's resistance to weight-loss. Have you ever been on a diet, happily losing weight, and the weight-loss stopped? Even though no one believed that you had been perfect, you knew that you had. This is a plateau.

Our bodies have a safety mechanism that helps to protect us from starvation. When you are on a diet that allows you to burn stored energy, your body senses starvation. Dieting is simulated starvation from your body's perspective. A thousand years ago, if you had not recently killed a buffalo, your body could chemically alter its metabolism and become more efficient. This efficiency helped you to survive until you had obtained food.

Minimum of Food Minimum of Options

If you are trying to burn off stored fat, this starvation response is unwelcome, but it's there. **All conventional weight-loss programs deal with a plateau incorrectly, if at all. They tell you to eat less. If you are already at a minimum of food, they are at a minimum of options**. If your metabolism has slowed to a thousand calories a day, the last thing you need is to eat less or to continue starving and not lose any weight. So, you eventually give up and gain your weight back.

Dieting Begets Dieting

In the March 9, 1995 edition of the *N.E.J.M.*, it was demonstrated that metabolism increases as people eat more and gain weight and decreases as people eat less and lose weight. The article stated, "This energy expenditure was not related to the degree of adiposity or fat. It was related only to the resting and non-resting energy needs of fat-free mass."[6] In other words, metabolism is hormonally or chemically altered by the body. This was one of many studies to confirm that metabolism does indeed attempt to adapt to caloric intake.

The "maintenance diet" of most conventional weight-loss programs condemns you to a perpetually lower metabolism. If you have lost weight in the past and tried to maintain it by marginally eating, you were perpetuating a lower metabolism. You were condemning yourself to a lifetime of dieting. There is a better way. I discovered a method for raising metabolism back to where it was before dieting, without gaining the weight back. I wrote about it over twenty years ago. I'll share it with you in a few chapters.

Chapter Review

*Conventional weight-loss plans are flawed because they condemn you to perpetual dieting.

*In spite of poor exercise and eating habits, most people very slowly gain extra weight.

*Pregnancy is an exception to slow weight gain and a good example that demonstrates how hormonal influences can alter metabolism.

*There are subtle influences which allow metabolism to adapt to eating or dieting.

*Past failures with weight-loss efforts should not influence a new decision based on new information. It was and is unreasonable to expect success with perpetual dieting.

CHAPTER III

OUR PAST AFFECTS OUR PRESENT

- **"Designing Women"**

- **Born to Lose**

- **Dieting Purgatory**

- **Been There — Done That**

- **They Call "This" Progress**

- **It's the Real Thing**

- **Turning Wheat into Sugar**

- **Deep-Fried Carcinogens**

- **Superficial Reasoning**

- **Trading Protein for Carbohydrates**

- **Oops!**

- **Chapter Review**

"Designing Women"

Man (or woman) was designed for survival. We have inherited these genes from our ancestors, and, although our genetics have served us well, we have not adapted well to "progress."

Early men were primarily hunter-gatherers, existing on protein and fats from animals, birds, and reptiles along with carbohydrates during the warmer months. During the winter months, dried meat was the major preservable resource.

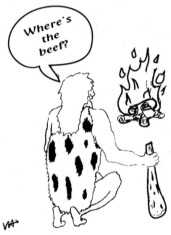

People, as most other mammals, ate well during the warmer months and gained extra body weight for nutrition and insulation to survive the winter. It's interesting that during the warmer months, carbohydrates were both abundant and that carbohydrates stimulate insulin. Insulin is the hormone that enables us to store energy in the fat cell.

It's also interesting that people lived almost exclusively on protein and fat during the colder months. This weight cycling for half of the year, with its high-protein, moderate-fat and low-carbohydrate diet, served them apparently quite well. How well did they live? Archaeologists actually determine the classification of a prehistoric society as hunters or farmers by the condition of their bones and teeth. If their bones are dense and long and the teeth are strong and not decayed, they are hunter gatherers. If their bones are frail and underdeveloped and their teeth are worn and decayed, they are agriculturists.[7]

Peter Brown, on page 6 of his article, "An Anthropological Perspective on Obesity," includes the following dietary chart:[8]

	Late Paleolithic	Contemporary American	Recommended
Protein	34%	12%	12%
Carbohydrate	45%	46%	58%
Fat	21%	42%	30%

What he does not recognize in the article is that almost all of the carbohydrate intake occurred about six months of the year. During the other months, fat and protein are almost exclusively consumed, to the exclusion of carbohydrates. This weight cycling allowed us to spend time each year losing the weight we had gained during the abundant months.

Weight cycling was reviewed by the N.I.H. with their National Task Force on the Treatment and Prevention of Obesity. They concluded, "There is no convincing evidence that weight cycling in humans has adverse effects on body composition, energy expenditure, risk factors for cardiovascular disease, or the effectiveness of future efforts at weight-loss."[9]

Born to Lose

We were designed to be in a fat-storing mode for periods of time and a fat-burning mode for others. Progress has allowed us to be indefinitely in a storing mode, preparing for the long winter that never comes. You must burn off the excess storage in a deliberate fat-burning mode as you were designed to do. Temporarily dieting is the price for overeating and under-exercising that caused you to store the excess fat. You will find that, if there is an end in sight, rather than a perpetual diet, it is a price you will more easily pay.

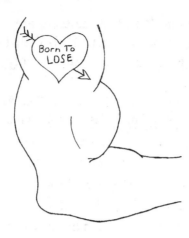

Dietary Purgatory

The conventional wisdom on dieting is that you remain in some neutral position. This perpetual diet is the primary reason people cannot achieve and maintain a weight-loss. While dieting, your body has the ability to adapt to a lower caloric intake, often before you lose all of the extra weight. You still maintain some or most of a previous weight gain but your metabolism has been drastically lowered. You are eating less and weighing almost the same. Does this sound familiar?

The previous chart shows that ancient man consumed more protein and less carbohydrate than that recommended by modern nutritionists. In the associated article, they establish that this higher protein consumption provided for a better quality of life. Peter Brown states, "Nearly everywhere it has been studied, the switch from food foraging to agriculture is associated with osteological evidence of nutritional stress, poor health and diminished stature."[8]

Nutritionists and dietitians recommend that we eat a diet that is mostly carbohydrates. They believe that the average American's consumption of eleven percent protein is adequate and that the lower our fat intake is, the better. They believe that dietary fat is responsible for our being fat. In fact, they want us to eat much like the ancient Egyptians.

Been There — Done That

Egypt is an excellent laboratory to analyze the high-complex carbohydrate, low-fat and low-protein diet that nutritionists claim will make us trim and healthy. Thousands of mummified remains from their golden-agriculture era allow us a window into their health. Their extensive written records describe their diet and their illnesses.

In the Nile valley, Egyptians were able to produce abundant crops of grain. They were able to store the grain so that they had an available supply of food. Processing of these complex carbohydrates were limited so that they retained a much higher nutrient value than our breads today. They had access to limited amounts of protein from cattle and fish, and their low-fat intake was almost exclusively the monounsaturated fat from olive oil. They must have been in perfect health, right?

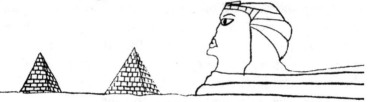

This must be where they got the food pyramid.

Thousands of mummified remains show a different picture. Mummification was commonly practiced. Wrinkles of skin in certain areas of the body show obesity as a common occurrence. Worn teeth and frail bones are typical of poor health. Atherosclerosis, or clogged arteries, in thirty-year-olds was rampant. Examination shows arteries that are plaque filled and calcified, as well as scarred and thickened, indicating high blood pressure. Heart disease was as prevalent as it is today. Their physical stature and length of life was limited.[10] Perhaps it's time to question the conventional nutritional wisdom of today. History does not have to repeat itself.

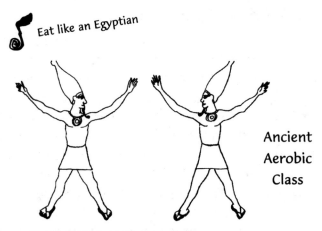

Eat like an Egyptian

Ancient
Aerobic
Class

They Call "This" Progress

No where in recorded history has there been more extreme changes in diet than we as Americans have experienced in modern times. The quantity of calories that arc available to us with the standard of living we enjoy, as well as refrigeration and variety, are unique in time. Our great-grandparents chose from only a dozen or so food items in an average week. Our modern grocery stores stock as many as 50,000 different items, almost all within the average consumer's budget. Eating has become a major recreation.

It's the Real Thing

The biggest culprit in my opinion is refined sugar. In the year 1900, the average American consumed about five pounds of sugar annually. According to The U.S.D.A., Economic Research Service, in 1992 the average American consumed one hundred and forty two pounds.[11] Around the turn of the century, Coke® was invented. Many people are drinking, five or six times each day, a glass of liquid that contains six to ten tablespoons of sugar. Consuming sugar stimulates the production of insulin, which starts the fat-storing processes our ancient genetics have programmed. This refined sugar has had all of its nutrients removed. It is pure energy whose excess is available for storage.

Sugar began to appear at the breakfast table for our kids. It's advertised as "part of a complete breakfast." What part is that? Isn't it really amazing that we are not heavier than we are?

Turning Wheat Into Sugar

Another culprit entered the picture about the time of refined sugar. We developed the technology to refine wheat and rice around the turn of the last century. Refining these grains eliminates the course roughage, which contains the fiber and many nutrients. Chromium, an essential trace mineral, is over 90% destroyed in the refining process. A chromium deficiency has been linked to diabetes. Diabetes was so uncommon in the year 1900 that it was around number one hundred on the list of common diseases in America. Today it is number five or six, at any given time. These refined grains are digested to glucose as quickly as table sugar. They evoke an insulin response, and their excess calories are available for storage just as quickly.

Deep-Fried Carcinogens

The third major change in our diet came with vegetable oils. We recently developed the ability to extract oil from seeds, abundantly and cheaply. Prior to the turn of the century, we consumed very little vegetable oil. Particularly with the advent of fast food, which is usually deep fried, we are consuming mostly polyunsaturated vegetable oils. These are the fats that are recommended by experts as "safe." These experts have had us run from butter and other molecularly stable saturated fats. We'll be talking about oxidation and free-radical damage later.

Superficial Reasoning

During the 1970s, dietitians and nutritionists (some of the same group that wants us to eat like ancient Egyptians) decided that fats were bad, and carbohydrates were good. They made this decision primarily for two reasons. The plaque that accumulates on arterial walls contains fatty deposits of cholesterol. They figured that, if you quit eating fat and cholesterol, you would have less disease-causing plaque in the arteries. The problem with this superficial thought was that cholesterol is only the final stage of this plaque. Consistent research demonstrates only a minor reduction of serum cholesterol with a low-fat diet. A lot goes on before cholesterol begins to adhere to the arterial walls.

Ask yourself why cholesterol doesn't build up on the walls of veins. It's present in the blood there, as well. The reason is veins do not have a muscular lining, as do arteries. Damage to the muscle tissue from free radicals, insulin, and other factors begins the plaque-building process with cholesterol as only the final stage.

Michael Oliver, Professor Emeritus at the National Heart and Lung Institute in London, released a shocking analysis at the First International Conference on Fats and Oils and Human Disease. He concluded that studies of people whose diets achieve the 30% goal of total fat intake show that the diet had virtually no effect on cholesterol levels.[12]

The other reason that fat was deemed bad was due to its calorie content. A gram of fat contains nine calories, whereas a gram of protein or carbohydrate contains only four calories. People were taught that fat in the diet becomes fat on the body. Of course, it's not that simple.

Trading Protein for Carbohydrates

In our panic to escape fat, we ran to carbohydrates. After all, you have to eat something. Since high-quality, animal protein contained fat, we also began to eat less protein. Since the 1970s, we have followed the "party line" of eating less fat and guess what? We are fatter than ever, and heart disease is rampant. According to the Department of Agriculture, in

1977 and 1978, Americans consumed 40% of their calories as fat. From 1994 through 1996 fat consumption went down to 33%.[13]

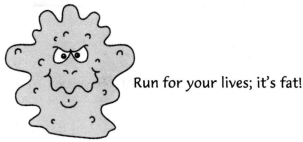

Run for your lives; it's fat!

Oops

Fat consumption dropped 17% while obesity increased by 25%.

A Dutch epidemiologist writing in the International Journal of Obesity, in 1995, pointed out that, as populations get fewer of their calories from fat, their waistlines nonetheless continue to grow.[14] **Walter Willet, chairman of the Harvard School of Public Health says, "The studies are clear. It's a myth that it's just the fat in your diet that makes you fat."[15]**

If a plumber's plumbing won't hold water you get a new plumber!

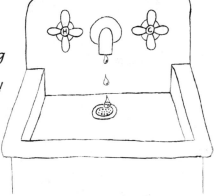

The number one vegetable in America today is the French fry. All those carbohydrates that we switched to are fried in oils or laced with fat. The only thing we really accomplished was to exchange protein for carbohydrate, or sugar.

Chapter Review

*People were designed to store fat in the warmer months, and carbohydrates enabled the process.

*During the winter, people were able to exist on protein and fat and burn stored energy safely.

*Progress has allowed us to be in a perpetual storing mode for the long winter that never comes.

*Diets do work if they are temporary and not high in carbohydrates.

*Too much of anything can be bad for you. Too much sugar, refined foods, and unstable oils can kill you.

CHAPTER IV

NUTRITIONAL REVIEW

- **We Are What We Eat**

- **Of First Importance**

- **The Skinny on Fat**

- **Carbohydrates Are Sugars**

- **Carbohydrate Addiction**

- **Glycemic Index of Foods**

- **Influence of Food on Insulin and Glucagon**

- **The Fiber Advantage**

- **Chapter Review**

We Are What We Eat

Let's review the basics on nutrition. The human body uses **protein**, **carbohydrate,** and **fat** from the diet to sustain tissue and to provide for energy. There are **water-soluble** and **fat-soluble vitamins** that are necessary to support body chemistry. There are **major minerals** that serve as electrolytes, structural components and chemical processors. There are **trace mineral**s that fill a variety of needs, and, as the body is composed mostly of **water**, that is an essential nutrient as well.

Of First Importance

Proteins are strings of amino acids that the body utilizes to sustain tissue, to build enzymes and other critical components, and to provide for energy. We need about ten to twelve essential amino acids. I say "about," because there is some debate. By "essential," I mean that the human body is unable to build these amino acids from others. In their absence, health is impaired.

Animal-derived protein provides all of the essential amino acids. Meat, cheeses, eggs, seafood, and poultry are good sources of complete protein.

Vegetables, grains, and nuts contain incomplete protein. These protein sources must be mixed and matched to consume all the essential amino acids if you are not eating animal protein.

The ancient Greeks recognized the significance of "protein" by the very meaning of the word, "of first importance."

Protein, during digestion, breaks down slowly into amino acids and enters the bloodstream. These amino acids flow throughout the body and provide the building blocks of tissue repair. They contain available energy, if needed, without overstimulating insulin. If you are not eating protein on a regular basis, the body will protect itself by utilizing amino acids from less essential muscle tissue and even vital organs.

If you burn up muscle tissue for energy, you lower your metabolism and disable your body in its ability to produce other essential components.

The minimum daily need for protein is from .5 to 1 gram per pound of body weight. There are about seven grams of protein per ounce of lean meat.

As people get older and have abused their digestive systems by poor food choices, their bodies produce less hydrochloric acid. Proteins are digested in an acidic environment. It's more difficult to digest the protein; therefore, you must eat more than the minimal amounts recommended. If you are strength training, you need even more. The previous generations that have programmed our genetics consumed a lot more protein and fared well.

The Skinny on Fat

Fats are available from animal as well as vegetable sources. Animal fats are considered saturated in that they are solid at room temperature. They have a more stable molecular structure. Vegetable fats are considered unsaturated and are liquid at room temperature. They have a less stable molecular structure. A third type of fats are the monounsaturated fats, such as olive oil. They are more stable than the vegetable oils and are considered to be healthier due to a lesser potential for oxidation and free-radical damage to cells.

The Mediterranean countries use olive oil almost exclusively. A high percentage of their diet is fat, but much of it is monounsaturated fat. It is believed that their low rate of heart disease, in spite of their high-fat diet, is a result of the type of fats they eat.

Margarine is an hydrogenated oil. Vegetable oil, such as corn oil, has hydrogen molecules forced into it. This allows the oil to become solid at room temperature. It looks and spreads like butter. The human body has trouble recognizing this man-made food, with its very unstable molecular struc-

41

ture. There is enormous potential for free-radical damage as it circulates throughout the body.

The Harvard Nurses Study confirmed that the nurses who ate margarine had a higher incident of cardiovascular disease than the nurses who ate butter.[16] Yes, it's true. Butter is better due to its stable molecular structure.[17]

Linoleic acid is an essential fatty acid that can be derived easily from many foods. The Omega fatty acids are now considered essential by many experts and can be derived from certain fish or fish oils. Fatty acids maintain the myelin sheath protecting nerves and are necessary to metabolize vitamins and provide energy.

Carbohydrates Are Sugars

Carbohydrates are essentially sugars. Fructose is the sugar from fruit. Sucrose comes from plants such as sugar cane or sugar beets. Lactose is the sugar present in milk. All carbohydrates are converted into glucose, which is the form in which your body can utilize them.

The glycemic index is a rating of how quickly a food is able to raise blood sugar. Pure glucose is the basis, with a rating of one hundred. The more fiber, protein, and fat a food contains, the lower its glycemic rating. These substances slow the digestion and absorption of carbohydrates. This is important because elevated blood sugar stimulates the production of insulin, the fat storage hormone.

An appropriate insulin response to a low glycemic food, allows blood sugar to rise slowly due to the slow absorption of carbohydrate. The body is then able to respond gradually with insulin. This appropriate response prevents the fat-storing mode and the other effects of too much insulin.

High-glycemic foods quickly raise blood sugar, stimulate a strong insulin response, and burn off quickly. The body then is left with too much insulin, which lowers blood sugar and leaves you hungry, light headed, and dizzy. The quickest relief is more sugar, and the cycle continues.

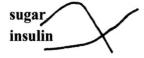

Carbohydrate Addiction

Carbohydrate addiction is finally being recognized as a biological factor in weight control. C. Everett Koop, M.D., former Surgeon General of the United States labels us "carbohydrate sensitive." Researchers have shown that up to 75% of overweight people are addicted to carbohydrates.[18] If you are a carbohydrate addict you may find that:

You have difficulty stopping once you've started to eat bread, pasta or other starches, snack foods or sweets.

After you've had a full breakfast, you get hungrier before it's time for lunch than if you had skipped breakfast or had only coffee.

You get tired or hungry in the mid-afternoon.

You have a tendency to put on weight easily, regularly, or on occasion.

Bread or other starches, snack foods, or sweets have been your diet downfall.

When you restrict your carbohydrates while dieting, you will find that you are hungry less often and have fewer food cravings. It's easier to stick with your diet even though the variety of food is limited. For a carbohydrate addict, "carbs cause you to crave carbs."

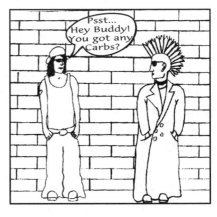

Glycemic Index of Foods

High Glycemic Food (Greater than 85)

Honey, Corn Syrup
Bagel, White Bread
Cornflakes
Raisins
Potato, (white, russet baked) 116
Corn

Moderate Glycemic Foods (60-85)

Spaghetti, Macaroni
Oatmeal
Banana, Grapes, Oranges
Rice
Yams 70
Baked Beans

Low Glycemic Foods (less than 60)

Apples, Cherries, Dates, Figs, Plums
Kidney Beans, Green Peas, Navy Beans, Red Lentils
Milk 44
Most nuts 15

Influence of Food on Insulin and Glucagon

TYPE OF FOOD	INSULIN	GLUCAGON
Carbohydrate	*****	no change
Protein	**	**
Fat	no change	no change
Carbohydrate & Fat	****	no change
Protein & Fat	**	**
High Protein & Low Carb	**	*
High Carb & Low Protein	*********	*

The previous charts demonstrate how the foods we eat affect the body's insulin or glucagon response. Both hormones are present in the blood at the same time. What drives the metabolism to store or burn is the dominance of one to the other.

When you look at the average American meal, you can see where the problems arise. We eat steak and a baked potato, a hamburger and french fries, lasagne, etc. Large amounts of carbohydrate with small amounts of protein cause the greatest insulin response.

Notice that fat raises insulin levels primarily in the presence of carbohydrates. It's true that fat is the raw material for cholesterol, but insulin runs the cellular machinery that actually makes it. If you reduce the level of insulin, the cells cannot convert the fat to cholesterol. If you reduce the amount of carbohydrate when you add the fat, you could see a reduction in serum cholesterol.

Glucagon is the fat-burning hormone. Notice that a high-protein, moderate-fat and low-carbohydrate diet will stimulate the production of glucagon. The body gets rid of fat by burning it and does not need the fat-cell building mechanisms of fluid retention and cholesterol production.

Fruits and vegetables that are primarily carbohydrates contain vitamins, minerals, phytochemicals, fiber, and beneficial nutrients that we are still discovering. These foods are definitely good for you. However, when you are in your fat-burning mode, it is difficult to eat a lot of carbohydrates and burn body fat. These sugars stimulate insulin and its fat storing properties. They inhibit glucagon and its fat-burning properties. They provide energy for the muscles but nothing to maintain the muscle structure which sustains metabolism.

When you are not in your fat-burning mode, complex carbohydrates are an important part of your foods. However, processed grains, such as white bread or rice, have almost no nutritional value and are converted to glucose faster than sugar.

By eliminating these processed as well as sugared foods and drinks, you'll spend a lot less time in the fat-storing mode.

When you are in a fat-burning mode, you find that protein meals satisfy longer and that you experience hunger less often. This contributes to the success of high-protein diets. You usually end up eating less calories because you're not hungry.

The Fiber Advantage

Fiber is the cellulose portion of plants that is not digested. Soluble fiber forms a gel-like substance which expands and moves slowly through the upper digestive system. This gives you a fuller feeling, that lasts longer. A study of young women who were given a high fiber, low fiber, and even lower fiber diet showed a difference in food absorption. Those with the lowest fiber absorbed 97% of their food. Those with the highest amount of fiber absorbed only 92.5%.[19]

According to David Heber, director of the Center of Nutrition at the University of California at Los Angeles, "Fiber moves food faster through the intestinal tract so that fewer calories are absorbed."[20]

Fiber-Nature's Broom

One recent study by the U.S. Department of Agriculture showed that consuming 24 grams of fiber a day blocks 90 calories.[20] The National Cancer Institute recommends 30 grams of fiber daily.[20]

Another study in 1994 comparing the diets of lean and obese men and women found the lean women's diet contained 45% more fiber than the obese women's diet.[21]

There are health benefits for fiber beyond weight control. Type II diabetics benefit from eating complex carbohydrates with higher fiber content. Fiber slows the absorption of sugar and allows for a slower, more appropriate insulin response, reducing their need for medication.[22]

Judith Marlett, a University of Wisconsin researcher says, "Soluble fiber drains cholesterol out of the blood."

A medical journal review compared the American Heart Association, low-fat, low-cholesterol diet with diets high in fiber. The American Heart Association diet lowered blood cholesterol only 3%. Fiber supplements decreased it by 16%. Oat bran or beans lowered cholesterol by 19%. Over the long term, studies showed a 25% reduction in LDL, the "bad" cholesterol, and increased HDL, the "good" cholesterol, by 10%.

A recent study showed that, among middle aged to elderly men, adding 10 grams of fiber to their diet resulted in a 20% decrease in heart attacks.

Fiber is a positive health factor in preventing the diseases of the bowel due to its water absorption properties. Stool that is soft, large, and moist moves through the intestine more quickly.

Colon cancer is the second leading cause of cancer death in the U.S. Numerous studies have linked a high-fiber diet with a lower level of colon cancer. They are speculating that it is the decreased time that carcinogens are exposed to the intestinal wall or that the cancer-causing elements are just diluted due to the increased bulk.

Diverticulosis, hernias, hemorrhoids, and ulcerative colitis are all associated with fiber levels in the diet.

Soluble fiber, which expands and forms a gel, is found in oat products, dry beans, lentils and barley. Insoluble fiber, which doesn't dissolve in water, is often referred to as roughage. This fiber comes from the outer hard shell of grains and is found in most fruits and vegetables. Bran, celery, green beans, green leafy vegetables, potato skins and whole grains are a good source.

Soluble and insoluble fiber work together, slowing the exit of food from the stomach when you want it to be slow. Then they speed the exit from the intestine and bowels when you want it to be fast.

Dietary Fiber in Foods

Food	Amount	Dietary Fiber (grams)
Asparagus	4 med spears	.9
Broccoli	1/2 cup	3.2
Cabbage, boiled	1/2 cup	2.0
Carrots, boiled or raw	1/2 cup	2.3
Corn, off the cob	1/3 cup	3.1
on the cob	1 ear	5.9
Lettuce	1/6 head	1.4
Potato, baked with skin	med	3.0
french fried	10	1.6
Apple, with peel	1 med	3.3
Banana	1/2 med	1.6
Cantaloupe	1/4	1.6
Grapefruit	1/2	.6
Orange	1 small	2.4
Raspberries	1/2 cup	4.6
Strawberries	1/2 cup	1.7
Cracked wheat bread	1 slice	2.1
Hamburger bun	1	1.2
Whole wheat	1 slice	2.1
All bran cereal	1/3 cup	9.0
Bran buds	1/3 cup	8.0
Raisin bran	1/3 cup	4.0
Popcorn	1 cup	.4

Chapter Review

*Protein foods are essential to health. Animal sources of protein are complete. Daily protein intake of .5 to 1 gram per pound of body weight is necessary.

*Fats have been poorly understood by professionals. Polyunsaturated and hydrogenated fats are unstable and can cause free-radical damage to cells.

*Carbohydrates have been promoted by professionals even though our annual consumption of refined sugar has risen from 5 pounds to 146 pounds. Carbohydrates stimulate the production of insulin with its fat storing properties and other health concerns.

*Many people are addicted to carbohydrates whereby their consumption leads to overeating and obesity.

*The fact that foods influence our biochemistry does not need to remain a mystery.

*Fiber was only recognized as an important nutrient as recently as the 1980s.

CHAPTER V

LIVING ON STORED ENERGY

- **Most Members Need Not Diet**

- **High Protein Opportunity**

- **Understanding Ketosis**

- **Back to Calorie Counting**

- **Test I Symptoms of Carbohydrate Intolerance**

- **Test II Carbohydrate Intolerance**

- **Test III Calorie Sensitivity**

- **Chapter Review**

Most Members Need Not Diet

Many members of Curves, women between the ages of thirty and eighty, have never strength trained or acquired the habit of exercise. When they begin to exercise with a complete program, their bodies respond quickly. Many have elevated metabolisms due to years of high-sugar consumption.

By eliminating sugar and starting an aerobic and strength training program, most of our members reach their goals without having to diet.

Yea!!!

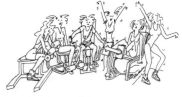

When It's Time to Diet

If you have more than twenty pounds to lose or yo-yo dieting has lowered your metabolism, you'll need to restrict food intake for a while. You want to go into your fat-burning mode.

Simply limiting calories would suffice if all foods had the same effect. If you restrict your protein calories, you may lose muscle as part of your weight-loss and lower your metabolism. If you eat mostly carbohydrates, your body will burn these sugars for energy rather than stored fat. You'll also have elevated insulin levels promoting fat storage and resisting fat burning.

High Protein Opportunity

Remember, **in the context of utilizing stored energy**, which is to maximize fat loss, to protect muscle and to sustain energy, I recommend a diet that is:

Higher Protein

Lower Carbohydrate

Lower Fat

There is a window of opportunity for the majority of people to take advantage of a high-protein diet with less restriction of calories. This program does not work for everyone. If you are one of the majority for whom it does work, there are advantages to this type of diet.

You might have heard of diets by Dr. Atkins, Dr. Stillman, or *Protein Power* by Drs. Eades. Millions of people have used their methods to safely lose weight. Their diets work because many of us can eat larger quantities of protein and even fat (in the absence of carbohydrates) without the excess being available for storage. Remember that it takes insulin to store fat and carbohydrate to stimulate insulin.

Our abuse of carbohydrates has caused many of us to lose our insulin sensitivity, and this creates a window of opportunity to utilize these methods of dieting.

The advantages of a high protein diet over calorie counting are:

You can eat more and still lose weight.

Protein burns slowly and gives us a steady source of energy and diminishes hunger.

A high intake of protein provides amino acids to sustain metabolically active muscle.

Fat in food is satisfying and prolongs the feeling of fullness.

The disadvantage of a high-protein diet is that you cannot cheat. As soon as you throw carbohydrates into the diet, your body is able to utilize and store the energy in fat and protein. Refer to the chart on the "influence of food on insulin and glucagon."

Understanding Ketosis

Ketosis is a by-product of losing weight on a high-protein diet. The human brain utilizes glucose as its primary energy source. In the absence of carbohydrate and glucose, your liver can alter fat so that it can be utilized as energy by your brain. These ketones are only partially burned and then excreted in urine, sweat, or breath. If you are trying to burn off stored fat, this incomplete burning of fat results in a faster weight-loss.

In her book, *The Nutritional Desk Reference*, Elizabeth Somers states that "Ketosis is an abnormal state."[23] Is it an abnormal state when we are in a fat-burning mode? I believe that ancient man spent half of the year in a state of ketosis. This state was designed to provide the type of energy that our body requires in the absence of carbohydrates.

Ketosis is often criticized because it is confused with ketoacidosis. The type I diabetic must be careful to maintain proper blood glucose levels so that their blood does not become too acidic. People with kidney or liver problems should consider a high-protein diet only under the advice of their physician.

Moderate ketosis is safe for people in good health as long as they drink adequate amounts of fluid to keep their kidneys flushed and get adequate nutrients to maintain their electrolytic balance.

Ketone testing sticks may be purchased from most pharmacies. Place the test stick in the urine stream, and it will turn purple if there are ketones present. This is one indicator that can show the loss of body fat while dieting.

Back to Calorie Counting

About 25% of people do not lose weight on a high-protein diet. Their bodies are able to utilize the energy available in protein and fats in the absence of carbohydrates. These people must restrict calories to burn stored body fat. They still need to eat higher protein, lower fat, and lower carbohydrates to lose body fat effectively.

Another 25% of people are moderately carbohydrate intolerant. They can enjoy the benefits of a high-protein diet temporarily, but then they must begin to restrict calories in order to continue burning stored fat.

The Institute For Nutritional Science has devised a sample of questions to determine if you are carbohydrate intolerant or calorie sensitive. Take the following three tests to determine your best method of dieting:

Test I Symptoms of Carbohydrate Intolerance

*Nervousness
*Irritability
*Fatigue and Exhaustion
*Faintness, dizziness, cold sweats, shakiness, weak spells
*Depression
*Drowsiness, especially after meals or in mid-afternoon
*Headaches
*Digestive disturbances with no apparent cause
*Forgetfulness
*Insomnia
*Needless worrying
*Mental confusion
*Rapid pulse, especially after eating certain foods
*Muscle pains
*Antisocial behavior
*Overemotional crying spells
*Lack of sex drive
*Leg cramps & blurred vision
*Shortness of breath, sighing and excess yawning
*Cravings for starch and sugar rich foods

Test II Carbohydrate Intolerance

1. You are more than 25 pounds overweight.
2. You have had a tendency to be overweight all of your life.
3. You have been overweight since you were very young.
4. You have a poor appetite and often skip meals.
5. You have food cravings that temporarily go away when starch or sugary foods are eaten.
6. There are foods that you feel you absolutely could not do without.
7. Your waistline is bigger than your hips.
8. Most or all of the symptoms associated with carbohydrate intolerance apply to you (Test I).

Test III Calorie Sensitivity

1. You had a normal body weight when younger but slowly gained weight after age 30.
2. You are presently overweight but by less than 25 pounds.
3. You have a normal appetite-get hungry at meal times.
4. You have few, if any, food cravings.
5. You have maintained the same basic eating habits all of your life.
6. You eat three meals per day.
7. You have gained a certain amount of extra body weight but seem to have tapered off (not continued to steadily gain more and more weight).
8. You have few or none of the symptoms associated with poor carbohydrate metabolism (Test I).

If you agreed with more statements on Test II, the carbohydrate-intolerance quiz, you should be successful on a high-protein diet. If you agreed with more statements on Test III, the calorie-sensitive quiz, you should restrict your calorie intake. If you agreed with a similar number on both, you can probably start with a high protein diet and enjoy its advantages, but you will need to restrict calories later to continue losing weight.

Chapter Review

*Many of our members can expect to reach their goals without having to diet.

*Dieting should be a temporary condition, where you go from being a food burning machine to that of a fat burning machine.

*High-protein and low-carbohydrate dieting works for most people.

*High-protein dieting allows you to eat more, have more energy, feel fuller longer, and protect muscle.

*The disadvantage of a high-protein diet is that you cannot cheat.

*Ketosis is a by-product of losing weight on a high-protein low-carbohydrate diet. Ketosis is often confused with ketoacidosis. Healthy people who drink adequate amounts of water and take supplements to maintain their electrolyte balance can safely lose weight with a low-carbohydrate diet.

*Many people can only lose weight by limiting calories. Carbohydrates need to be limited so that the production of insulin, the fat storing hormone, is not overstimulated.

*Take the three tests to determine your best method of dieting.

Curves®

CHAPTER VI

HORMONAL INFLUENCES

- **Power Behind the Throne**

- **Counting Carbs**

- **Meeting Glucagon**

- **Master Hormones**

- **Survival Mechanism**

- **Prevailing Metabolism**

- **Homeostasis**

- **The Real Set-Point**

- **Starvation Hormones**

- **Chapter Review**

Power Behind the Throne

There are thousands of books that tell you the foods you can or cannot eat in order to lose weight. There are hundreds more that tell you how to exercise. There are just a few that teach you about the hormonal responses that actually control fat burning or storage. This "power behind the throne" will be a key to your success.

The most powerful of these hormones is insulin. Insulin is produced by the pancreas in response to a rise in blood sugar. Insulin's job is to lower blood sugar levels. It accomplishes this by transporting the glucose into muscle cells to be used as energy. What cannot be used by the muscles is then taken to the fat cells for storage.

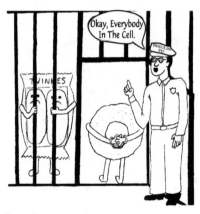

Counting Carbs

If you are trying to burn stored energy with a low-calorie diet that is 60% carbohydrate, you will stimulate the production of insulin. If these carbohydrates are bagels or rice, they burn off quickly and leave you with too much insulin and low blood sugar. You'll feel starved, and it will be difficult to not eat. You also will not have the energy to exercise.

Remember, carbohydrates stimulate the insulin response, and insulin is necessary for the storage of energy as fat. Do you see a problem with high-carbohydrate diets?

Meeting Glucagon

Glucagon is the opposing hormone to insulin. Glucagon makes energy available from the fat cells. As your blood sugar lowers, glucagon replenishes energy needs by facilitating the release of energy from stored fat. With our extraordinary intake of carbohydrates over the last twenty years, our bodies would hardly recognize glucagon. It's time to get acquainted with the fat-burning hormone.

Master Hormones

Let's look at the roles of the master hormones, insulin and glucagon.

Insulin	Glucagon
• lowers elevated blood sugar	• raises low blood sugar
• shifts metabolism into a storage mode	• shifts metabolism into a burning mode
• converts glucose and protein into fat	• converts protein and fat into glucose
• converts dietary fat to storage	• converts dietary fats to ketones for energy
• removes fats from blood and transports to fat cells	• releases fat from fat cells and makes it available for energy
• increases the body's production of cholesterol	• decreases the body's production of cholesterol
• makes the kidneys retain excess fluid	• makes the kidneys release excess fluid
• stimulates the use of glucose for energy	• stimulates the use of fat for energy

Survival Mechanism

We know that when we go on a diet that allows us to live on stored energy, our bodies respond. We are designed to become more efficient when we are living on stored energy.

As a survival mechanism, this is a wonderful thing. When we are trying to burn off stored energy, it's not.

One of the ways that our bodies become more efficient is that they produce lypogenic enzymes when we are dieting. "Lypo" means fat and "genic" means building. These enzymes facilitate the storage of fat. They allow the body to eek out the most energy from foods and resist the utilization of fat stores. The opposing lypolytic or fat "breakdown" enzymes facilitate the utilization of fat from storage.

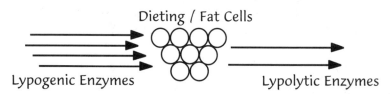

Dieting / Fat Cells

Lypogenic Enzymes   Lypolytic Enzymes

We know from research at Cedars-Sinai hospital that the human body will begin to increase production of lypogenic enzymes within seventy-two hours of dieting.[24] This "window of opportunity" will enable you to gauge your weight fluctuation. Seventy-two hours is the length of time you can diet and not restimulate the production of starvation hormones.

Prevailing Metabolism

A broader response to dieting is something I call "prevailing metabolism." I believe that your body responds to behavior. The body tries to maintain homeostasis or "like state."

Homeostasis

Homeostasis is a normal objective of many of the body's systems. PH and fluid balances are examples of carefully maintained processes of homeostasis that are necessary for survival. A law of physics states that a body in motion tends to stay in motion until acted upon by an outside force. Resisting change is natural.

The Real Set-Point

The body's set-point is actually determined by homeostasis. The body resists change.

Example: Your metabolism is 2500 cal/day. You need to lose twenty pounds of body fat. You gained ten of those pounds with a pregnancy and the other ten pounds over several years at a half of a pound per month. You went on a diet and lost twenty pounds, didn't exercise and ate 1000 cal/day with nominal protein intake.

Results: Up to eight pounds of your lost weight could be muscle, a couple of pounds of water, and the rest body fat.

Consequences: The lost muscle lowered your resting metabolism by 400 cal/day. The lost fat even lowered metabolism a small amount. Hormonally, your body responded to the simulated fast (diet) by becoming more efficient. Your metabolism has lowered to 1500 cal/day.

Choices: In the past you had two. You could go back to eating as little as 2000 cal/day and you would quickly regain your lost fat, but not the muscle. Sound familiar? Your second choice would have been to stay on a maintenance diet of 1500 cal/day forever because that's where your metabolism had been set. How were you at that?

Is it any wonder that you have not been successful at the weight-loss game? Let me give you a new scenario.

Example: Your metabolism is 2500 cal/day. You need to lose twenty pounds of body fat. You gained ten pounds with a pregnancy and the other ten pounds over several years at a half a pound a month. Now you begin exercising with a program that includes both aerobic and strength training efforts. You restrict your calories to 1500 /day but eat adequate protein to sustain muscles and limit carbohydrates to avoid overstimulating insulin.

Results: You lose twenty pounds. Three pounds are water,

but you have lost twenty pounds of fat. You have gained three pounds of muscle.

Consequences: The three pounds of muscle gained require an extra 150 cal/day. However, your resting metabolism has hormonally responded to the simulated fast (diet) and has gradually lowered to 2000 cal/day.

Choices: In the next chapter, you will learn how to readapt metabolism to a higher caloric intake but not regain your weight. You do this by eating and allowing a small gain. You diet just long enough to lose the small gain but not long enough to restimulate the production of starvation hormones. Time will allow the saturation of starvation hormones to dissipate, and your body will become stabilized at this new weight. Your metabolic rate will increase and become less efficient due to the quantity of food that you are eating.

Your second choice is to continue exercising and burn an extra 500 cal/day, which increases your metabolism to 2500 cal/day and allows you to eat normally. The best choice is to do both. You can eat 3000 calories a day if you protect and increase muscle tissue, exercise, and raise metabolism by eating rather than by "maintenance dieting."

In essence, you reset your set-point by getting to your new weight and staying there long enough. There are genetic influences that affect weight gain that you cannot control. The strongest influence is homeostasis, which you can control.

Starvation Hormones

From the body's perspective, dieting is a simulated period of starvation. We know that it can become more energy efficient when sensing starvation. It resists change by slowing the loss of fat. You may know this as a plateau.

The body, trying to maintain homeostasis, produces these "starvation hormones." These hormones increase the energy efficiency of the body by lowering metabolism.

What about when we are habitually eating too much? The body responds hormonally by raising metabolism and reducing our energy efficiency. By resisting change, we don't quickly become immobilized by morbid obesity. It takes a long time and a lot of hard work to gain an extra hundred pounds. In our frustration, we fail to acknowledge the magnificence with which we are made.

Perpetual dieting adapts the body to a perpetually lower metabolism by lowering the prevailing metabolism. Eating raises the prevailing metabolism. These influences are subtle but important.

Prevailing Metabolism while dieting

Prevailing Metabolism while eating.

How do you eat to keep your metabolism high without weighing too much? Allow me to introduce you to the Heavin Formula for metabolic change.

Chapter Review

*Effective weight-loss requires more than the calories consumed minus calories burned approach.

*The master hormones, insulin and glucagon, respond to your diet and control whether you are burning or storing energy.

*Our bodies are able to respond to famine (dieting) by becoming more energy efficient.

*Cedars-Sinai hospital demonstrated a seventy-two-hour window before our bodies begin to lower metabolism.

*Prevailing metabolism is the real set-point. The human body resists change with a process of homeostasis.

CHAPTER VII

PERMANENT RESULTS WITHOUT PERMANENT DIETING

- **The Heavin Formula**

- **Phase I**

- **Higher Protein/Low Carbohydrate**

- **Calorie Version**

- **Phase I**

- **Phase II**

- **Phase III**

- **Window Of Opportunity**

- **Flawed Conventional Wisdom**

- **Note 1**

- **Note 2**

- **Chapter Review**

The Heavin Formula

I wrote a book in 1978, *The Sweet Joy of Sugar Free Living*. I outlined what I called "The Heavin Formula for Metabolic Change." Working with thousands of women, I had discovered a method that was simple and effective in utilizing the hormonal factors of weight control. Your use of these hormonal factors will enable you to finally control your weight. Using these factors will give you the ability to lose weight when you need to. You will know when it is time to diet and when it is not. After losing the desired weight, you will be able to stabilize at the new weight and raise your metabolism. Then you will deal with the small weight gains before they can add up.

Phase I

I believe that it is important to be able to lose weight when you need to. This ability as well as your confidence will be a tool that is necessary to control your weight. The choice is clear — control your weight or your weight will control you. I recommend a fairly restrictive diet for the first one to two weeks of your weight-loss program.

In the following chapters, you will find meal plans for your preferred method of dieting.

Higher Protein/Low Carbohydrate

Unlimited protein, moderate fat, 20 grams of carbohydrates

Calorie Version

40% or more of your foods comprised of proteins

No more than 60 grams of carbohydrates

1200 total calories per day

On either plan

*You may add a Curves shake

*You must drink 8, 8 oz. glasses of water each day

*As your food choices are limited, you need to take a good vitamin and mineral supplement such as Curves Complete. This will assure that you have any missing nutrients and electrolytes.

*You may have coffee, tea, diet drinks, and artificial sweeteners

Most women lose between 5 and 10 pounds during the first two weeks. Some of this is water weight. It is important that you replenish these fluids by drinking adequate amounts of water.

If you have less than 20 pounds to lose, you can spend just one week on Phase I, otherwise two weeks.

The objectives are to get you off to a great start and to have a tool that will allow you to lose weight when you need to. Because you have adequate protein and calories and are strength training with the Curves workout program, you should not lose muscle.

Phase II

After one or two weeks on Phase I, you need to increase your food intake.

*If you have been on the higher-protein version, raise your grams of carbohydrates to sixty per day.

*If you are counting calories, increase your caloric intake to sixteen hundred, but keep your grams of carbohydrate at sixty per day.

You should expect to lose a couple of pounds per week. Most people can safely lose body fat at that rate.

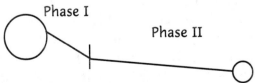

There are 3500 calories in a pound of fat. If you are increasing your daily activity by 500 calories and decreasing

your food by 500 calories, the math says that you should burn 7000 calories from storage, or two pounds each week. If you are eating 1000 calories per day less than normal, you could lose three pounds of body fat each week.

A higher-protein diet advantage is that you are incompletely burning fat to produce ketones. This additional caloric deficit will speed your weight-loss.

You will stay on Phase II as long as you are losing weight, or until you reach your goal.

If you have to spend more than a month or two dieting, your prevailing metabolism will lower. This is your plateau. Conventional dieting advice is to hang in there or lower your calories until it is unhealthy. Rather than lower your calories to an unacceptable level, you should move on to Phase III and raise your metabolism. When your metabolism is sufficiently higher, you will go back to Phase I and II until you reach your ideal weight.

If you need to lose more than one hundred pounds, you will repeat this cycle several times. There's nothing worse than to be on a strict diet and not to see any results.

Phase III

When you reach your ideal weight you have successfully burned your excess fat storage. The next objective is to raise your metabolism to where it was before you started dieting but not gain your weight back. Remember, dieting stimulates the production of starvation hormones. Eating stops the production of these hormones. You need to begin eating to raise your prevailing metabolism.

There is no "maintenance diet." You start eating normally again even rewarding yourself for what you have accomplished. You do have to weigh every day. You will gain weight. Don't panic: you know how to lose weight when you need to. You now are confident that you can lose weight when you need to. Allow yourself a weight gain of a few pounds. I call this your "high" weight. You will gain these three pounds in just a couple of days. It is mostly water weight as your body rehydrates. Discount normal monthly weight fluctuations.

As soon as the scale shows your high weight, go back on Phase I for a couple of days. Your strict Phase I diet is a guaranteed method of losing those few pounds quickly. You will lose the water weight and the small amount of fat that you have gained.

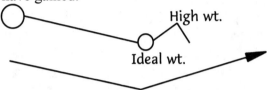

Prevailing Metabolism

At your ideal weight, begin eating again. You will find it takes a little longer to reach your high weight. What is happening is that the starvation hormones are slowly diminishing. Your body is raising its metabolism to adjust to the higher caloric intake.

The key is to diet just long enough to lose the small amount of weight you gained but not long enough to re-stimulate the production of starvation hormones.

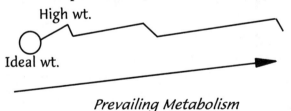

Prevailing Metabolism

Window of Opportunity

Cedars-Sinai hospital research demonstrated that lypogenic enzymes begin to rise after seventy-two hours of dieting.[24] This indicates that your body begins to prepare for a fast after this period of time. This is why you only allow a

71

small weight gain. You can only diet for two or three days without restimulating the production of starvation hormones.

Flawed Conventional Wisdom

Conventional programs teach you to stay on a maintenance diet to retain a weight-loss. This causes the continual production of starvation hormones and perpetuates a lower metabolism, and, as a result, these programs force you to diet forever.

With our program, you will eat more and diet less, raising your prevailing metabolism while maintaining your weight-loss. **Notice that over a thirty-day period of time, you will diet six or eight days and eat twenty or more days.** This allows your body time to diminish the starvation hormones and adapt to eating. The length of time it takes to raise your metabolism depends on a number of variables. If you have been dieting for a long time, you will need to diminish a greater saturation of starvation hormones

Most people stabilize at their new weight within a month or two.

Once you have increased your metabolism to a reasonable level, you only need to deal with the small amount of weight gain that caused you to become overweight. For the average overweight person, that is about a half of a pound a month. How long does it take you to lose a half of a pound?

Can you diet two days a month if you can eat reasonably well the other twenty-nine days for the rest of your life?

Anne Fletcher, in her book, *Thin for Life*, studied 160 people who had lost at least twenty pounds and kept it off for three years. She says that the vast majority of these people kept it off by never allowing a weight gain of more than five pounds.[25]

Dr. Thomas Wadden, M.D., director of Syracuse University's Center for Health and Human Behavior says,

"Reversing small weight gains as they occur is the single most important skill that patients fail to learn in conventional weight-loss programs."[26]

You now have something reasonable to grasp. For the first time in your life, you can have the hope and means to control your weight and protect your health.

Note 1

If you have sabotaged your metabolism by yo-yo dieting or restrictive eating, you may have to raise your metabolism before you can safely lose weight. When I met my wife, Diane, she was doing two hours of aerobic classes daily. Her weight was 115 lbs. on a 5'7" frame. She saw herself as fat and was eating less than 800 calories per day. Her metabolism had adjusted to this extremely low calorie intake in spite of a high level of activity. She could eat as few as 1200 calories and still gain weight.

She needed to gain ten pounds of weight, most of it as muscle. She also needed to be able to eat normally without continually gaining. Diane needed to raise her prevailing metabolism.

She spent two months on Phase III. She ate 2000 calories a day and quickly gained up to 125 lbs. At 125 she ate 1000 calories for two or three days and lost back to 122 lbs. She ate again until she weighed 125 lbs. It took longer and longer to regain those few pounds. After two months, she could eat a normal diet of 2000 calories daily without gaining weight.

Note 2

If you cannot lose weight eating less than 1500 calories, you must begin with Phase III and raise your prevailing metabolism. Spend a month following the plan in Phase III. Weigh every day. Eat two to three thousand calories per day. When you gain three pounds, diet for two or so days to lose what you have gained. Begin to eat again. You will find that you regain those few pounds more slowly as the month goes by. Having raised your prevailing metabolism to two or three thousand calories a day, you are ready to safely lose weight.

Most women who use the Curves workout system can lose up to 20 pounds of body fat without having to diet. By burning an additional 300 to 500 calories per day and performing resistance exercises to protect and increase muscles, they can expect significant and lasting change. As they begin to invest in their health, their eating habits improve, and they will have the energy to be more active.

If they have more than 20 pounds to lose or have sabotaged their metabolism with perpetual dieting, they need to diet to reach their goal. Restricting calories is too simplistic. Choosing the best method of dieting, high protein or calorie counting with a limit on carbohydrates, will provide for the most efficient loss of only body fat.

Dieting lowers prevailing metabolism. The Heavin Formula will raise your prevailing metabolism. People can achieve "permanent results without permanent dieting."

Chapter Review

*For over twenty years, I have been expecting researchers to announce that they discovered what I had put together through observation and trial and error.

*The Rockefeller study affirmed the raising and lowering of metabolism in response to feast or famine.[6]

*Cedars-Sinai hospital confirmed the production of lypogenic enzymes at seventy-two hours as the window of opportunity to diet.

*Conventional wisdom still teaches that a calorie is a calorie, and you must perpetually diet to maintain a weight-loss.

*Learn how to lose weight quickly as a tool to control your weight.

*Use the best method of dieting for your biochemistry.

*Once you reach your desired weight, begin to eat so that you can raise your metabolism, but limit your gain to a few pounds.

*Diet just long enough to lose the small weight gain but not long enough to cause a starvation-hormone response.

*Once you have stabilized at your goal weight, deal with the small amount of gain that caused the problem.

Curves

CHAPTER VIII

NUTRITIONAL SUPPLEMENTATION

- **The Body's Building Blocks**
- **NPK**
- **Pesticides**
- **Chronic Disease Predicted**
- **The Importance of Vitamins**
- **Perimeter Shopping**
- **Medical Journals**
- **RDA**
- **Results of Studies**
- **Vitamin E**
- **Chromium, Glucose Tolerance, and Diabetes**
- **Arthritis**
- **A Woman's Needs**
- **Curves Complete**
- **Curves Integrated**
- **Curves Essential**
- **Curves Herbal Fem**
- **Curves Weight-loss Shake**
- **Chapter Review**

The Body's Building Blocks

The human body is really amazing. Most things around us wear out faster the more they are used. Our bodies wear out faster the less they are used. Exercise keeps all of the systems of the body operating at peak efficiency. The cellular machinery that constantly replaces worn tissue enables this wonderful process.

Nutrients are the building blocks of this cellular machinery. If you are not getting all of them in your diet, you will eventually experience the consequences. **Given enough time, a nutritional deficiency will ultimately manifest itself as disease.**

Progress has allowed us to leave the fields and to rely on large scale farming to provide nutrient rich foods for our sustenance. The price of progress has been an epidemic of chronic disease, but it need not be.

The soils of the earth contain many of the nutrients as minerals. When a plant grows in these soils, they take up minerals which enable their own healthy growth. Plants alter the molecular properties of minerals. They coat them with substances that allow our bodies to recognize them as food. They alter their electromagnetism to a negative charge which our positively charged bodies can better absorb. When we eat the plants, we ingest the minerals that are the building blocks of a healthy body.

NPK

In the earlier part of this century, we adopted a national farming policy of NPK fertilization. Experts found that you could put just three minerals back into the soil and grow a large, healthy looking plant. Nitrogen, phosphorus, and potassium were the only nutrients being replenished in our soils. For almost seventy years, we have been farming the same soils and only replenishing three minerals. Long ago, the minerals that were originally in the soil were depleted.

Many areas of the country are lacking certain minerals to begin with. The mineral selenium, which has been shown to protect heart muscle, does not naturally occur in one-third of the soils in the U.S. Refining of grains has further removed many of the minerals from the foods we eat.

Pesticides

During the 1940s, crops which had been fertilized with NPK became pest infested. Bugs were designed to eat dying, unhealthy plants. Even though the appearance and bulk of these farm products could be sustained by three minerals, they were mineral deficient. Pesticides then had to be used to protect these unhealthy plants from bugs. Inexpensive farming methods led to pesticide-coated and mineral-deficient foods. These problems still exist.

Chronic Disease Predicted

In the U.S. senate, during the 1930s, it was predicted that, if we maintained the current farming practices, in fifty years, we would see the largest epidemic of chronic disease in history.[27] These diseases included diabetes, heart disease and arthritis. This prediction has obviously come true.

The Bible says, in Genesis, that we are made from the dust of the earth. You can do a chemical analysis of the ashes of a human body and guess what? You will find the minerals which come from the soil. There are a lot more than three of them. A deficiency of any one of them can eventually show up as disease.

The Importance of Vitamins

Vitamins, which are usually produced by the plants that we eat, are better understood. After all, most of our mothers told us, "Don't forget to take your vitamins." However, we have a long way to go.

If you are counting on eating an orange from the supermarket to attain your vitamin C, you should expect 180 mg. That orange in all likelihood was picked green before it had a chance to form vitamin C in the last stage of ripening. It sat in cold storage until your grocer called in his order. The wholesaler went in and sprayed a ripening agent (complete with an orange-flavored scent) to ripen the orange. That fresh looking and fresh smelling orange quite possibly has no vitamin C.[28]

Perimeter Shopping

Cooking, processing, freezing, and canning destroys vitamins that are in foods. We should eat as much as possible of our foods in their natural state. Raw vegetables and fruits are much better for us. You should shop only on the perimeter of your grocery store and then only carefully.

Medical Journals

Here are several professional journal reports on vitamins and minerals:

*"At least 20-30% of U.S. adults ingest less than 60 mg of vitamin C per day." Lancet, March '98[29]

*"One-third to one-half of 70 plus year old Caucasian U.S. women have lost 25% of their femoral bone mass and reached the osteoporotic state." Nutrition and the MD, Aug., '97[30]

*"Intakes of Zinc, Calcium, Vitamin A, Vitamin B6 and Folate were frequently less than 2/3rds of the RDA." Journal of the American Dietetic Assoc., Nov., '97[31]

*"These data demonstrate that the average daily intake of Chromium from self selected diets is well below the minimum suggested safe and adequate intake." Am J Clin Nut, June '85[32]

*"These prevalence correspond to app. 700,000 toddlers and 7.8 million women with iron deficiency; app. 240,000 toddlers and 3.3 million women have iron deficiency anemia." JAMA, March '97[33]

RDA

The RDA "recommended dietary allowance" and the newer term RDI, "reference daily intake," are virtually the same in their amounts of vitamins and minerals. They are slightly above the minimal amount of a nutrient necessary to avoid disease. I don't know about you but I'm interested in the amount necessary to attain optimal health.

In the *American Journal of Clinical Nutrition* it stated, "Substantial evidence indicates that intakes greater than the RDI of vitamins and minerals reduce the risk of certain diseases." '97[34]

If a medical doctor or dietitian claim that there is no evidence that vitamin and mineral supplements have been proven to prevent disease, they are correct in the context of the minimal amounts recommended by the RDI. Almost all the major nutritional studies of disease treatment and prevention are at higher levels. For example:

Nutrient	RDI	Clinical Studies
Vitamin E	30 IU	400-800 IU
Vitamin A	5,000 IU	10,000-50,000 IU
Vitamin C	60 mg	1-3 gm
Chromium	120 mcg	200-500 mcg
Selenium	70 mcg	200 mcg

Results of Studies

Here are the results of some of these studies:

"**Vitamin E** can lower the risks of heart attack, as observed in a double-blind, placebo-controlled study on 2002 people with coronary atherosclerosis." Lancet 1996; 347(9004): 781-786[35]

Nutrient Supplemented	% Decrease in risk of Heart Attacks	% Decrease in other Heart Disease Events
Vitamin E 400-800 IU/day	77%	47%
Placebo	No Significant Decrease	No Significant Decrease

Chromium, Glucose Tolerance and Diabetes

"Chromium functions by increasing the activity of insulin and therefore reducing the amount of insulin required to control blood sugar and related processes. It is important to keep insulin at low levels to prevent secondary signs of diabetes." Bilo. Trace Elem Res. 1992[36]

Arthritis

"It is suggested that . . . glucosamine sulphate should be considered for the basic therapy of primary or secondary osteoarthrosis, mainly because it restores articular function to a certain extent." Current Medical Research & Opinion. 1980:7[37]

When was the last time your cardiologist told you to take vitamin E because it decreased the risk of heart attacks by 77%? When did your doctor last ask you if you were taking your chromium for diabetes? When did your rheumatologist last recommend glucosamine?

A Woman's Needs

With our focus on women's fitness, it was necessary to find solutions for their unique nutritional needs. After all, we are exercising in a way that causes the body to protect itself from chronic diseases such as osteoporosis, arthritis, heart disease, and diabetes. If the building blocks necessary for cellular maintenance and repair were not available in the diet, we had to find them some other way.

What does the body really need?
*10-12 amino acids
*3 fatty acids
*16 vitamins
*70+ minerals
*Phytonutrients
*Heavy-hitting antioxidants

These nutrients need to be in the most absorbable form possible and in the proper ratio to each other. Synergy is critical for safe and effective supplementation because nutrients work together.

Curves Complete

We could not find a well formulated multivitamin and mineral supplement designed for women. So we went to the experts, who created Curves Complete to provide the essential nutrients that are needed for a woman's optimal health. Curves Complete has the following advantages:

*All natural vitamins, no synthetics
*The proper ratio of nutrients to assure synergy
*An acidic base to enhance absorption
*Plant sourced trace minerals, recognizable by the body
*Major minerals in chelated form for best absorption
*Liquid form to allow for colloidal or small particle size
*Specific nutrients for a woman's needs

Curves Integrated

Curves Integrated is for joint support. It contains the substances glucosamine and chondroitin sulphates along with MSM, trace minerals and vitamin B-6 that have been shown to help maintain the integrity of joints.

Curves Essential

Curves Essential is our calcium supplement. It includes the form of calcium and minerals which were proven in a double-blind study to actually restore bone density.

Curves Herbal FEM

This supplement is an herbal blend designed to support and maintain a woman's biochemistry during life's transitions.

Curves PMS Formula

This supplement helps to alleviate the symptoms of PMS by helping to balance the hormonal changes that occur during a woman's monthly cycle.

Curves Weight-loss Shake

We created a delicious drink with our Curves Weight-loss Shake that is rich in nutrients including soy protein with isoflavanoids, the natural estrogen. Each shake contains twenty grams of protein and has only twenty grams of carbohydrates. Its herbal blend speeds the digestive process and helps to detoxify the body. It comes in chocolate and vanilla and uses no artificial sweeteners or sucrose. When you have to diet, it is a wonderful reward that will help you to stay motivated.

Chapter Review

*Nutrients are the building blocks of a healthy body.

*A deficiency of any nutrient can eventually manifest itself in disease.

*The soils of America no longer contain the original nutrients.

*We have been replacing only three minerals, NPK, for the last seventy years.

*Unhealthy plants require pesticides, which have contaminated most of our foods.

*Rampant chronic disease was predicted over seventy years ago based on the deficiency of minerals caused by our farming methods.

*Vitamins are usually made by the foods we eat, but processing, cooking, and canning destroys many of them.

*The medical and nutritional journals are validating the need for supplementation, but health professionals have been very slow to respond.

*The recommended dietary allowance "RDA" is just over the minimal amount of a nutrient needed to prevent certain diseases.

*Studies are consistently showing that adequate doses of vitamins are able to fend off disease.

*Supplements must have certain qualities to be useful. We are not designed to eat soil.

*Out of necessity, we formulated and developed supplements to provide for the unique needs of women.

Curves®

CHAPTER IX

CHRONIC DISEASE

- **What Your Doctor May Not Know**

- **The Medical Model in America**

- **Free Radicals**

- **Hyperinsulinemia**

- **Osteoporosis**

- **Type II Diabetes**

- **Arthritis**

- **Hypertension, or High Blood Pressure**

- **Heart Disease**

- **Back Problems**

- **Obesity**

- **Chapter Review**

What Your Doctor May Not Know

We expect our doctors to be experts in all the areas that affect our health. Why does it seem that they have very little information about nutrition?

Dr. Kenneth Cooper is a leading force in the utilization of nutrition in the medical field. In his book, *Advanced Nutritional Therapies*, he explains "Like most physicians, I am something of a Johnny-come-lately to the nutrimedicine scene. I was never offered a course in nutrition in medical school."[38]

If the medical journals are reporting the nutritional studies, why aren't doctors learning about nutrition? Generally doctors are too busy working to keep up with the journals they receive.

In fact, doctors get much of their post-education information from pharmaceutical companies. They are provided with materials and samples from salesman on a regular basis. They scan the studies and prescribe the product. Pharmaceutical companies are not motivated to produce and promote nutritional supplements because they are not patentable. There is no profit motive for them.

A recent cover of *Fortune Magazine* stated, "America's Most Profitable Business, It's Pharmaceuticals." It continued with, "The pharmaceutical industry says it spends 15% of sales on R&D." Fortune found out that the industry spends up to twice that much on marketing.[39]

There is a greater concern than just missing out on inexpensive natural treatment that would often help our bodies to heal themselves. In an article in *U.S. News and World Report*, Jan 9,'95, it was written, "Statistics show that up to 2 million patients are hospitalized each year and as many as 140,000 die of side effects or reactions related to various prescription drugs."[40]

In defense of doctors, we expect immediate relief. You don't usually get that with nutrition. We accept from them the following method of treatment.

The Medical Model in America

Diagnose

Prescribe Drugs

Perform Surgery

As a result, the symptoms of disease are often treated rather than the cause. Most chronic diseases have at their cause a nutritional deficiency. The human body is a biochemical factory. According to *Senate Document No. 264*, "Any upset of the balance, any considerable lack of one or another element, however microscopic the body requirement may be, and we sicken, suffer, shorten our lives..."[27]

I believe that American doctors are dedicated, caring people who work hard at what they do. They are the best diagnosticians in the world, and they save many lives with miraculous innovations. However, in the area of nutrition, you need to educate yourself and your doctor.

On a daily basis, Curves deals with the chronic diseases of thousands of women. These women are taking a proactive approach to disease. A complete approach must include not only exercise but nutrition and supplementation. Along with the care of their doctors, they are doing all that they can to protect and restore optimal health. The most common chronic diseases that affect women are:

- Osteoporosis
- Diabetes
- Arthritis
- Hypertension & Heart Disease
- Back Problems
- Obesity

This chapter will define these conditions and describe the effects of exercise, nutrition and supplements that help protect and restore health.

Free Radicals

An understanding of free radicals and their potential to cause disease is essential in our battle to prevent most chronic diseases. Chemically speaking, free radicals are atoms or groups of atoms that are highly reactive with other substances due to the fact that they have at least one unpaired electron. This causes them to bond with other compounds and hence cause damage to a wide variety of tissues in the body. Free radicals can attack cells and cell groups, playing a devastating role in virtually every chronic degenerative disease.

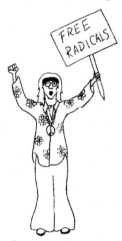

Free radicals can form under a variety of circumstances. Pollution, chemicals, drugs, stress and even aging all produce free radicals primarily through the action of oxygen. The interaction of oxygen, superoxide, peroxide, or other substances can affect the cellular material with which it comes into contact. These substances have available electrons that emit a small electrical charge when reacting with other substances.

This reaction can alter the genetic code of cellular reproduction. Cells replicate by duplicating their DNA code and transferring it to the new cell. The original cell divides but the new cell is different than the original. This new cell will continue to divide and duplicate itself with the new genetic code. This process is called genetic mutation.

It is believed that almost all cancers, arthritis, adult onset diabetes, most heart disease and dozens of other "mysterious" diseases have as part of their causes, genetic mutations. An arterial muscle cell that has been genetically altered by free radical damage can aggressively duplicate and damage the arterial wall. This lesion along the arterial wall can begin the plaque-building process that results in atherosclerosis. The unchecked growth of cancerous cells have been linked to the mutations caused by free-radical damage.

Any damage to a cell membrane that results in the reduced capability of that membrane to transport nutrients, oxygen, water, and excretion of wastes can damage surrounding tissue. Rheumatoid arthritis and type II diabetes with its loss of cellular sensitivity to insulin may be caused in part by free-radical damage of tissue.

Remember the Harvard Nurses Study which found that the nurses who had eaten margarine rather than butter had more heart disease?[16] Polyunsaturated oils which are hydrogenated are extremely unstable. These unstable molecules have tremendous potential for free-radical damage, particularly in the arterial walls. Monounsaturated oils like olive oil or natural fats like butter are far more stable and less likely to cause free-radical damage.

The body has natural defenses to free-radical damage. This complex network of antioxidants attacks free-radicals and protects membranes, nucleic acids, and other cellular constituents from destruction. This system is dependent upon nutrients such as vitamin E, C, and A, beta carotene, selenium, zinc and others.

We have the worst onslaught of poisons in our environment in human history. Pesticides, pollution, chemicals, smoking, and many other modern factors have increased the potential for disease. Science has discovered powerful free-radical fighters with greater protection potential than those previously known. These "heavy hitting" antioxidants include substances such as grape seed extract and Coenzyme Q10. Lycopene, found in tomatoes and concentrated in tomato sauce, has been found to be ten times more powerful than beta-carotene. This is believed to help explain why prostate cancer occurs less frequently in the southern Mediterranean countries where tomatoes are a staple.

Hyperinsulinemia

In previous chapters you learned that insulin is produced in response to a rise in blood sugar. A diet high in carbohydrate demands a high production of insulin. In 1900 the average American consumed about five pounds of sugar annually. In 1992, we consumed one hundred and forty-two pounds.[13] Seventy-five percent of overweight people are carbohydrate addicts and carbohydrate intolerant.[18] Many of us are in a constant state of hyperinsulinemia as a result of our carbohydrate-saturated diet.

Some of the consequences of hyperinsulinemia may be:

Diabetes

*A loss of cellular sensitivity resulting in the need for greater and greater amounts of insulin production in maintaining safe blood glucose levels.

*The resulting condition of adult-onset diabetes when the body is no longer able to sustain a higher production of insulin.

Heart Disease

*Insulin is a growth hormone which can cause muscle cells in the arterial walls to grow and narrow the vessels, contributing to atherosclerosis.

*Cholesterol levels and LDL, the bad cholesterol, are increased in response to the growth mode stimulated by insulin.

*Insulin fuels an increase in the production of triglycerides, a form of fat that circulates in the blood.

Hypertension

*Insulin causes the kidneys to retain fluids, which increases blood volume.

*Insulin stimulates an adrenaline-like hormone that increases heart rate and constricts blood vessels, similar to the fight-or-flight response.

Obesity

*Insulin facilitates the storage of energy in the fat cells.

Notice that the cause of many of the chronic diseases of this century can be traced to hyperinsulinemia. Gerald Reagan, MD., professor of medicine at Stanford University dubbed insulin resistance disorders, "Syndrome X." He associates all of the above disorders as having a common cause.[41]

Dr. DeFronzo, MD., head of the Diabetes Division at the University of Texas, Health Science Center at San Antonio, uses the following diagram of an iceberg to illustrate the effects of hyperinsulinemia.[42]

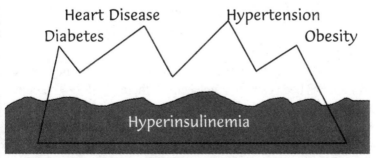

Many doctors are treating only the symptoms of these diseases. The only way to reduce the level of insulin in your body is through diet. Break the sugar and refined food habit. Don't be afraid to eat ample amounts of protein and moderate fats.

Osteoporosis

Osteoporosis, or "porous bone," is characterized by reduced bone mass and increased susceptibility to fractures. It occurs more commonly in men under age 45 and in women after age 45.[43] It affects an estimated 15 to 20 million Americans. This weakening of the bone is responsible for 1.3 million fractures in older people each year and accounts for between 30 and 50 thousand deaths. One out of every four women over the age of sixty experience a bone fracture due to osteoporosis, and seventeen percent of those who sustain a hip fracture die within three months.[44]

After reaching its peak, bone mass can decline as we age. Bone rebuilding is a process that requires certain nutrients and responds to certain activities. The bones serve as a reservoir for calcium homeostasis. When there is either too little calcium in the diet or a lack of digestive acids for absorption, the bones will give up their calcium. If you have elevated calcium levels in your blood test and do not have a condition that can explain it, you almost always are deficient in calcium. Other biochemical needs take priority over bone density such as the blood, heart, muscular system, nervous system, and hormonal system. The calcium removed from the bone is very alkaline and remains in the blood as the body attempts to acidify it. This explains the high serum level of calcium in the midst of a deficiency.[44]

The medical response to osteoporosis in postmenopausal women has been estrogen replacement therapy, ERT. The objective was to stop or delay the loss of bone density that occurs during the first few years following menopause. Progesterone was included in the hormone therapy so as to not increase the risks of certain cancers. They have now discovered that HRT increased the risks for stroke, heart disease and breast cancer to an unacceptable level. ERT is a poor choice in the effort to prevent osteoporosis. In premenopausal women, doctors generally recommend milk, vitamin D and calcium carbonate (hard to absorb, but cheap).

Resistance exercise or strength training is a behavior that stimulates the body to protect and increase bone density. Activities that include jumping, high-impact aerobics, jogging and running should be performed with caution.

The Health and Nutrition Examination Survey found that 50% of all females age 15 and older consume less than 75% of the RDA of 1200mg of calcium and that 75% of women over 35 consume less than the RDA of 800 mg.[45] To make matters worse, older women often have reduced digestive acidity from a lifetime of eating processed and dead foods. Calcium absorption requires an "acidic" environment. When you take Tums® to get your calcium, you are taking an "antiacid." Do you see a problem with this?

The first study to actually demonstrate a restoration of lost bone density was performed at the University of California by Strause and Saltman, *Journal of Nutrition*. 1994.[46] In a double blind, placebo-controlled, two year study on fifty-nine postmenopausal women, they found:

Nutrients Supplemented	% Gain or Loss in Bone Density
1. Placebo	3.52% Loss
2. 25 mg zinc, 5mg manganese 2.5 mg of copper	1.89% Loss
3. 1000 mg Calcium	1.25% Loss
4. 1000 mg Calcium + zinc, manganese & copper	**1.48% Gain**

Note: The calcium was citrate and malate, not carbonate.

1. Women should have their bone density checked by age forty. If the density is lower than 85% of expected density for their age, hormone replacement therapy, HRT may be considered. Alternatives to HRT are the natural estrogens found in certain foods such as soy, wild yams, corn, apples, carrots, barley and oats.

2. Women need to consume 1000 to 1500 mg of calcium daily. This is difficult to do without supplementation. If bone

loss has already occurred, the form of calcium and trace minerals which have demonstrated restoration should be used. (See preceding study.) Vitamin K, in heavy concentration, is found in bone and should be included with a full-spectrum nutritional supplement.

3. Whenever possible, it's best to get your nutrients from foods. Dairy products are high in calcium and vitamin D. Broccoli and kale are vegetable sources of calcium, and most people can attain vitamin D from thirty minutes of sunlight each day.

4. Exercise regularly, including load bearing activities.

Type II Diabetes

Diabetes is characterized by reduced insulin secretion or reduced sensitivity to insulin. Non-insulin dependent diabetes mellitus, NIDDM, is the most common form, affecting 90% of all diabetics. It typically occurs in adults who are overweight. Diabetics are essentially hyperglycemic (too much sugar). They are unable to control their blood glucose levels. Either their pancreatic beta cells are no longer able to produce adequate insulin or their tissues have become desensitized from years of too much insulin. Too much sugar in the blood can damage tissues in the body and lead to blindness, amputation, and heart disease, among other problems.

Even though genetics increases the chances of developing Type II diabetes, it is almost always preventable. It takes years of dietary abuse and overconsumption of sugar and refined foods before hyperinsulinemia takes its toll. The body is ultimately unable to produce the ever increasing amounts of insulin that the desensitized cells require.[47]

If you already have diabetes, it is imperative that you seek your doctor's guidance when beginning an exercise program or altering your diet. The medical regimens for treating diabetes are oral medications, insulin injection, and dietary modification. Review the diet that your doctor has given you. If it is printed by the Eli Lilly corporation (world's largest insulin manufacturer),[48] or the Mayo clinic, notice that they can be in excess of 60% carbohydrate.[49] Considering that a diabetic has difficulty keeping his blood sugar level down, doesn't it seem odd that you would be advised to eat mostly sugar-producing foods? Ask your doctor for an explanation.

Exercise has long been considered beneficial in treating or preventing diabetes. Aerobic and strength-training activities provide benefit through weight control, lowering of blood cholesterol and lipids, and improving insulin receptor sensitivity. Diabetics beginning to exercise should:

1. Check their blood glucose frequently.
2. Work closely with their doctor to determine the right insulin dosage.
3. Carry a rapid-acting carbohydrate.
4. Avoid exercise during the peak of insulin activity.
5. Don't inject into the primary muscles that will be used during the workout.
6. Take good care of their feet.
7. Omit supplements such as chromium without your doctor's participating.

Pre-diabetics can often prevent diabetes by reducing their dietary intake of sugar and sugar producing foods, losing weight and exercising. Without large amounts of carbohydrates in the diet, your body should be able to maintain adequate insulin production. Much of the receptor sensitivity can be reacquired.

Many studies have shown that the minerals chromium and vanadium will restore insulin sensitivity.[50] Chromium has long been considered essential in the metabolism of carbohydrates. More than 90% of chromium is destroyed in the refining process of grains.[28] According to the Nutrition Center of the U.S.D.A., more than 50% of Americans are deficient in chromium. The following conclusions were stated regarding chromium and vanadium.

"Chromium functions by increasing the activity of insulin and therefore, reducing the amount of insulin required to control blood sugar and related processes. It is important to keep insulin at low levels to prevent secondary signs of diabetes." Biol Trace Elem Res. 1992.32[51]

"These results indicate that 3 weeks of treatment with vanadyl sulfate improves hepatic and peripheral insulin sensitivity in insulin resistant NIDDM humans." Journal of Clinical Investigation. 1995: 95[52]

Self Health by Dr. Steven Whiting is an excellent book to help determine the appropriate levels of these and other supporting nutrients.

Consider these facts that since the year 1900:

*Our average annual sugar consumption has gone from 5 to 146 lbs.

*We began the refining of grains to "one step from sugar."

*Metabolically essential minerals such as chromium were processed out of grains.

Is it any wonder that diabetes has moved from number 100 to number 6 on the list of common diseases in America?

Arthritis

The two major categories of arthritis are osteoarthritis and rheumatoid arthritis. Osteoarthritis afflicts eighty-five percent of sufferers and rheumatoid arthritis about fifteen percent. Osteoarthritis is characterized by a deterioration of the joint. Rheumatoid arthritis is characterized by bouts of swelling within the joint and is more common in women. Both may progress to a loss of cartilage and connective tissue through repeated inflammation and irritation of the joint.

Arthritis is a chronic disease of this century. It was so rare in the year 1900 that, if you sought a specialist, you would have had to go to New York City. It is estimated that currently one out of every twenty people over age thirty-five suffer from arthritis.

The medical regimen for arthritis includes NSAIDS (non-steroidal antiinflammatory drugs), corticosteroids, anti-virule drugs, and joint replacement. For the most part, these treat the symptoms rather than the underlying cause. They reduce joint swelling and pain but with side effects that may worsen the condition.

Certainly, one of the causes of arthritis is free-radical damage to the joint components. Free radicals have been shown to erode the cartilage which serves as a shock absorber within the joint. Our modern toxic environment has contributed to the buildup of these poisons within the cartilage and synovial fluid. The deterioration of bone and cartilage within the joint is not usually a result of normal wear and tear. Given the proper nutrients and exercise, our joints are designed to maintain themselves. Calcium deficiencies and over-cooked processed foods are common factors with arthritis. Rheumatoid arthritis is sometimes associated with a virule infection. This can also be attributed to free radicals and toxins which provide the virus an available environment.

The cartilage within the joint is the focal point of osteoarthritis. It serves to absorb shock as well as to reduce the friction of bones rubbing against each other. This cartilage is much like a sponge. It has tremendous water-holding properties and is said to be ten times more slippery than ice on ice. There are no capillaries or circulation of blood within this cartilage. Nutrients and oxygen are taken in and waste products are removed by the up and down "squishing" of movement. This is why exercise can be an important part of joint health. Trauma, free radicals, infection, or missing nutrients may damage this cartilage and start the process of deterioration.

In the book, *The Arthritis Cure,* by Jason Theodosakis, M.D., you will find an informative approach to arthritis. He cites numerous studies which show that the substances glucosamine and chondroitin often help restore the joint cartilage and its qualities. He includes the following studies:

"In a double blind study, looking at 80 patients in Milan, Italy, all suffering from severe established osteoarthritis, participants were given 1.5 grams of glucosamine sulfate or a placebo, with the following results.

*The group treated with glucosamine experienced a significantly greater reduction in overall symptoms (73% versus 41%).

*It took only 20 days to reduce the symptoms by half in the glucosamine group.

*A full 20% of the glucosamine treated group became completely symptom free, compared to none of the 40 patients on the placebo."

They examined the cartilage of the glucosamine treated group following the study and found, "they looked strikingly similar to healthy cartilage."

In another double blind study conducted in Argentina, in 1987 comparing the effects of chondroitin sulfates with two groups of 17 having severe knee osteoarthritis. One group received a daily injection of 150 mg of chondroitin sulfates plus 500 mg of aspirin 3 times a day for 20 weeks. The second group received a placebo injection and the aspirin. After 20 weeks, 13 of the 17 receiving chondroitin injections experienced an improvement in pain, while only 2 of the 17 in the placebo group enjoyed pain relief.

Dr. Theodosakis states, "Working together synergistically, glucosamine and chondroitin sulfates stimulate the synthesis of new cartilage while simultaneously keeping the cartilage-busting enzymes under control."[53]

Exercise provides several benefits in the prevention and treatment of arthritis. The "squishing" of the cartilage from exercise, helps the cartilage to acquire oxygen and nutrients and dispose of wastes and toxins. A load bearing activity stimulates the body to protect and increase bone density. Movement and stretching assist the joint in maintaining freedom of movement and range of motion. Strong muscles can provide better support for joints.

It is a good idea to eat natural nutrient rich foods and remove processed, overcooked, free-radical producing foods from your diet. Taking a full spectrum supplement, including a quality calcium product will help assure that the essential nutrients for joint integrity are available. Glucosamine and chondroitin sulfates should be taken based on the exciting results of research and use. You should be patient. Most people who benefit from these nutrients find that it takes at least a month or longer before they feel better. Not everyone is helped by these substances, but they are relatively inexpensive and have few if any side effects.

Ask your doctor to get involved with your efforts to fend off or treat this painful, scary disease. Your approach should include a full arsenal of options aimed at the underlying cause rather than just the symptoms of arthritis.

Hypertension, or High Blood Pressure

As many as 50 million Americans have chronically elevated high blood pressures greater than 140/90 mmHg or are taking antihypertensive medication. Hypertension is related to the development of coronary artery disease, atherosclerosis, stroke, aortic aneurysms, and congestive heart failure. Hypertensive individuals are at three to four times the risk of developing coronary artery disease and up to seven times the risk of stroke.

When I am teaching a group of people, I ask who has high blood pressure. Then I ask them why they have it. Most people can't answer because their doctor doesn't usually know. I think that most people should have a good idea of the cause.

Stress management has become a common theme during

my lifetime. The stresses of daily life impose physiological changes on the human body. The "fight-or-flight" response is an inherited mechanism that contributes to our survival. Our bodies prepare for fight or flight by producing hormones such as norepinephrine which cause blood vessels to constrict to allow oxygen to get to muscles more quickly. The heart begins to pump faster, and, with constricted vessels, blood pressure rises.

You might have noticed these feelings after having been scared suddenly. Your face was flushed, and you felt a rush. In our hectic world, many of us are in a constant state of stress, which induces a perpetual state of fight-or-flight response. The medical regimen for hypertension induced by stress can include drugs that relax the stress response. These drugs have among their side effects personality change, expense, and lifetime need and mostly treat the symptoms rather than the cause.

Doctors have long recognized the benefits of exercise for lowering stress-induced hypertension. Exercise works by creating a controlled stress environment. Your body responds to the stress of exercise by constricting blood vessels and increasing heart rate. By limiting heart rate to a target zone, you safely create a stress response which conditions your body to a higher stress level. The results are that the minor daily events which formerly caused the stress responses are less able to cause them. You condition your body to not be stressed by the small things.

Another stress relieving mechanism resulting from exercise is the body's production of endorphins. These hormones naturally relax you and lower blood pressure. The euphoric feeling from exercise can be attributed to these substances.

Hypertension can be caused by hyperinsulinemia. A lifetime of too much insulin's circulating in the blood can affect blood pressure in several different ways. Insulin is a growth hormone which can stimulate the growth of arterial muscle cells. These muscle cells which line the arterial wall enlarge and narrow the artery. Since cholesterol serves as a part of the structure of all the cells in our bodies, the growth mode of insulin stimulates the liver to produce cholesterol and the LDL which transports it. LDL cholesterol is available to contribute to the plaque-building process in the artery. This narrowing is further aggravated by calcification of the arterial wall and a loss of elasticity. The narrow and rigid artery restricting blood flow forces the heart to pump harder which increases blood pressure.

Insulin causes the kidneys to maintain a higher sodium balance in the blood and as a result, higher blood volume. This higher volume of blood in circulation results in hypertension. Diuretics work by forcing the kidneys to get rid of a higher amount of sodium than they normally would. They get rid of this sodium by jettisoning fluid, which lowers blood pressure. Another option in reducing blood volume would be to lower insulin levels through nutrition.

Insulin also increases the levels of norepinephrine in the blood. As previously described, this substance constricts blood vessels and increases heart rate and elevating blood pressure in these scarred and thickened narrow blood vessels.

Some people have a genetically predetermined sensitivity to sodium. If salt intake influences your blood pressure, you should limit it.

*Hypertension is a dangerous condition and should be closely monitored and treated carefully by your doctor.

*As you begin to exercise and make dietary changes, work closely with your doctor to adjust medications.

*Initially, keep your target heart rate at 50% of maximum heart rate and don't be in a hurry.

*Keep in mind the title of a recent book, *Don't sweat the small stuff and it's all small stuff.*

Heart Disease

Cardiovascular disease is the leading cause of death in the western world. Ninety percent of heart disease is coronary artery disease, or CAD. The arteries that supply blood to the heart can narrow, calcify, and ultimately cause a heart attack. Heart disease in America is a recent phenomenon. It was so rare that the first department of cardiology in an American hospital was not opened until the 1930s. Coronary arteries suffer from the same effects as we previously discussed in all arteries. The consequence of diseased coronary arteries can be a loss of the blood flow which is the life support of heart tissue.

The plaque-building process that narrows arteries is not a result of too much cholesterol in the diet. If cholesterol is the problem, why doesn't it stick to the walls of veins? Something must cause cholesterol to stick to the walls of arteries. The difference between arteries and veins is the smooth muscle walls that line the inside of arteries.

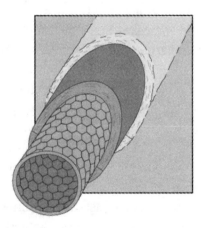

These muscle cells are exposed to free radicals which can alter their DNA. As these mutated cells reproduce, they are attacked by the body's defenses and lesions can occur. These lesions attract fibrin for repair, and the sticky fibrin can attract calcium and other substances in the blood. The final substance is usually cholesterol which gets all the blame.

An incredible study demonstrated that 400 to 800 mg of vitamin E taken by patients with coronary atherosclerosis, "resulted in a 77% decrease in the risk of heart attacks and a 47% decrease in other heart disease events!" Lancet 1996; 347(9004): 781-786[54]

The antioxidant effect of vitamin E is believed to be particularly effective in protecting the arterial muscle walls from the damage of free radicals. When was the last time your cardiologist called you and said, "You aren't going to believe this but you can reduce your chances of a heart attack by 77% with an inexpensive, safe vitamin!"

The standard diet for atherosclerosis is a diet low in fats except for vegetable oils (unstable, free radical forming). Angioplasty is a surgical procedure where a balloon-like device is inserted into the artery and inflated. The artery is enlarged, and the plaque is compressed against the arterial wall. Coronary bypass surgery is an invasive procedure where the chest is cracked open, and a vessel borrowed from the leg is sewn in to bypass the clogged coronary artery. Both angioplasty and bypass surgery are temporary and are required again in a few years. They prolong life but treat only the symptoms rather than the cause of heart disease.

*Prevention of heart disease can be aided by eliminating all vegetable oils except olive oil.

*Unstable polyunsaturated or hydrogenated vegetable oils contain the potential for tremendous free radical damage.

*Keep fat intake below 30%, but eat natural fats such as butter.

*Eat adequate protein and complex carbohydrates. Eliminate sugar, refined grains, and processed foods from your diet.

*Full-spectrum nutrition including antioxidants will help

protect the arterial wall from free radical damage.

*Exercise will keep the heart muscle strong and stress levels down.

*Stop smoking and eliminate the toxins in your environment and diet.

Back Problems

Lower back pain, LBP, accounts for 10% of all chronic health conditions in the U.S. and 25% of days lost from work. LBP has been labeled the most expensive benign health condition in America representing one half of all disability compensation payments annually. Four recognized causes of LBP are herniated discs, a trauma to the back, one vertebrae sliding forward on the vertebrae below, and degenerative disease.

LBP is often associated with an imbalance of strength and flexibility of the lower back and abdominal muscles. Poor flexibility in the hamstrings and hip flexor muscles are common. Many physicians believe that the major cause of LBP is simply physical deconditioning.

The muscles are designed to provide the structure and support of the body. Long bones and vertebrae serve as levers. If the muscles are not strong and firm, vertebrae can twist and turn and cause muscle spasms which begin a cycle of discomfort. A chiropractor can often realign vertebrae that are "subluxated" or misaligned. However, until the muscular support is in place, treatment will only be temporary.

It is believed that ninety-five percent of women over age sixty-five will have arthritis in their lower back. Proper nutrition, including joint-support nutrients, strength-training exercise, stretching, and chiropractic treatment when necessary might prevent much of this suffering.

*An individual with LBP should begin to exercise after obtaining their doctor's approval, including limitations and guidelines.

*Strengthening exercises for the lower back and abdominal muscles will aid in proper support.

*The Curves workout includes strength training for muscles in the neck, upper, and middle back as well as the abdominal and lower back muscles.

*Stretching the hamstrings (back of upper thighs) and hip flexors (front and top of legs) keeps the muscles from pulling forward or backward on the spine.

*Avoid unsupported lifting, twisting, lifting both legs in a prone position, rapid movements, or hyperextending.

Obesity

Most of this book deals at least indirectly with obesity. We have shown that you can overcome this dangerous condition. Don't let the past or the dismal success rate with conventional programs discourage you.

Use everything available in this battle, and you can be successful.

*Enlist your doctor's help to assure that your health needs are met by your diet and exercise.

*Set a reasonable and exciting short-term goal for weight-loss, eg. size 20 by Christmas.

*Create an environment that will allow you to be programmed for success. Enlist the support of family and friends, and tell everyone that you are losing weight. Put pictures of you at your best on the refrigerator door and on your bathroom mirror.

*Bad habits and good habits both take about a month to acquire. Work through the discomfort of starting an exercise and diet program. Soon, you will be uncomfortable when you don't exercise.

*Commit yourself to your Curves program. Surrounding yourself with other people who have the same goals is very important.

*Exercise at least three days a week and include all five components. Strength training will protect muscles and increase metabolism. Aerobic exercise will burn extra calories and condition the body for fat-burning metabolism. Exercise will give you a sense of accomplishment and replace the gratification you once felt while eating.

*Dieting should be a temporary condition, where you go from being a food-burning machine to a fat-burning machine. When you reach intermediate goals, you should increase your metabolism by following Phase III of our program. Don't stay on a strict diet when your weight-loss has stopped.

*While dieting, limit the sugar producing foods so that insulin levels will not prevent the accessibility of fat stores for energy.

*Be sure to eat adequately so that you will not lose lean tissue or put your health at risk.

*In prayer seek the power of Him who created us with the strength and mind necessary to overcome food addiction and inactivity.

Chapter Review

*The medical model in America treats illness rather than wellness. Chronic disease is often avoidable with proper nutrition and exercise.

*Carbohydrate addiction leads to hyperinsulinemia in many people. This may contribute to the higher rates of diabetes, heart disease, hypertension and obesity.

*Osteoporosis prevention and treatment requires a load-bearing activity, proper nutrition and the correct calcium supplement.

*Type II diabetes is almost always preventable. Pre-diabetics must work to reacquire insulin sensitivity.

*People with either type of arthritis must control their weight, strengthen muscles, stretch regularly and protect joint cartilage.

*Exercise is an effective method of lowering blood pressure.

*Cholesterol is only the final product in the plaque-building process. Proper nutrition and exercise may prevent heart disease in most people.

*Back problems are often the result of poor muscular support.

*The treatment of obesity requires burning stored energy (body fat). Once metabolism has adapted to the caloric deficit, it must be raised to maintain results.

Curves®

CHAPTER X

THE PSYCHOLOGY OF CHANGE

- **What's New?**

- **Embracing Change**

- **The Human Mind**

- **Attitude**

- **Goals**

- **Be Your Own Best Friend**

- **Steps In The Right Direction**

- **The Greatest Power**

- **Chapter Review**

*"For what I want to do I do not,
but what I hate, I do."*
— The Apostle Paul, Romans 7:15

We have all experienced the frustration of falling off some wagon, so why is it we cannot will ourselves to change our behavior? How do we acquire the habit of exercise and stick with a diet? We are going to answer these questions and devise a plan for change. **We are going to embrace change.**

What's New?

The Past Need Not Predict the Future

Let's begin with a reasonable assessment of our past experiences with exercise, dieting and weight-loss. From a physiological perspective, we may have been faced with exercise options that were doomed from the start because strength training was omitted from the regimen. We have learned that exercise must be complete; it must contain not only aerobic exercise and stretching but strength training as well. We now know that strength training protects and prioritizes muscle tissue while we are trying to lose weight.

Lose Fat Not Muscle

In the past, if you were dieting and doing some type of aerobic activity, it is likely that up to 40% of the weight lost was in the form of lean tissue. Muscle is metabolically active tissue, so a pound of muscle burns up to 50 calories per day at rest. If you lost 20 pounds, chances are 8 of those lost pounds came from your muscle mass. That means you lowered your daily metabolic rate by up to 400 calories. You set yourself up for failure.

Become Effective at Burning Fat

If you had no exercise regimen, you never experienced the physiological changes that allow your body to effectively burn fat. As your muscles burn energy from exercise, they become better at accessing energy, particularly the energy stored as body fat. The more active we are, the better our body burns fat stores.

No More Plateaus

We have learned that limiting calories lowers metabolism, yet conventional dieting requires that you limit calorie intake. The Rockefeller study demonstrated that as your body accesses stored energy due to actual starvation, fasting or dieting, a survival mechanism kicks in. Hormones are produced which allow your body to operate more efficiently. This survival mechanism is helpful to our species, and has allowed us to survive famine, long winters, and other hard times. But when we're trying to burn off energy that has been stored (body fat), this hormonal response becomes a great disadvantage. This is the reason weight-loss slows and a plateau is reached on any diet.

Perpetual Dieting Perpetuates a Low Metabolism

Conventional weight-loss methods also fail because they require you to stay on a diet forever. These may be called maintenance programs, but in truth they are perpetual diets. We now know that perpetual dieting perpetuates a low metabolism. Is it any wonder we have failed in the past? Don't despair, because we now have a method to raise metabolism.

Increase Your Metabolism

Our new definition of DIETING is that of a temporary condition whereby a food burning machine becomes a fat burning machine. Our goal is to spend a period of time safely and effectively burning off energy that has been stored (body fat). When you reach your goal or hit a plateau, you will deliberately raise your metabolism back to pre-diet levels. Once you have raised your metabolism, you will have to deal with about a half-pound of weight gain per month, on average. How many days of dieting does it take you to lose a half-pound? You may have to diet two days per month for the rest of your life, but you can eat normally the other twenty-nine days of the month.

If you have more weight to lose, you will cycle through Phase I and II more than once, until you reach your goal or hit a plateau. There will be no more futile efforts at trying to lose weight when metabolism is too low for success.

Let's review what we have learned:

* Strength training protects and prioritizes muscle tissue, and increases the body's energy requirements.

* Exercising while trying to lose weight conditions the body to access and burn stored body fat rather than just use the energy from the foods we eat.

* Perpetual dieting lowered our metabolism and past dieting methods required that we diet forever to maintain weight-loss because we did not have a means to raise metabolism without regaining weight.

* The Phase III plan allows us to raise our metabolism to pre-diet levels without regaining weight, and ensures that we are able to maintain weight-loss or lose more weight on Phase I and II.

"Insanity is doing the same thing over and over again and expecting different results."
— Albert Einstein

Embracing Change

To paraphrase Scott Peck in *The Road Less Traveled*, people change due to one of three reasons:

- They have spent adequate time in despair and frustration with their lives or circumstances.
- They have hit rock bottom.
- They learn that they can change.

Chances are that you have begun weight-loss programs due to despair or a feeling of hitting rock bottom. You may have begun the Curves program for these same reasons. This emotional foundation is very unreliable, and will increase your chances of failure. The reason for this is that when you begin to see progress, your motivation diminishes. You feel less despair after losing only a few pounds, so you have less motivation following small successes.

A rational plan provides a much better foundation for your efforts to change. Motivation increases and becomes more reliable as you learn that you can change. You will not depend on moods to move you forward. You will depend on a rational plan of action and choose change every day.

Character

Change involves moving out of your comfort zone. Yes, you are going to experience discomfort. Growth in any area of your life always requires moving out of that zone where we hide ourselves away, and we learn through suffering. I'm not talking about real pain here, I'm talking about pushing yourself physically so your muscles will get stronger and your heart will strengthen. I'm talking about eating less so your body will burn fat stores. Eating less and exercising more will tax your body and your self-discipline. You must get comfortable with being uncomfortable. **This is a key to success**.

"That which doesn't kill us makes us stronger."
— Friedrich Nietzsche

Dream Weaving

I have a passion for flying. I fly my own jet and compete as a hot air balloon pilot. Last year I decided to learn to fly helicopters. Helicopters are different than other aircraft. It is said that they're ten thousand parts all trying to separate. Like a bumblebee, they're not supposed to be able to fly. Every appendage is critical when flying a helicopter. The right hand is controlling the stick which moves you forward, backward and sideways. The feet are keeping the aircraft from spinning to the right or the left. The left hand controls the collective that keeps you in the air, allows climbs and descents, and controls the throttle for power.

My first six hours of helicopter training were humiliating and filled with fear. I had stepped right out of my comfort zone. I felt like I wouldn't be able to do it, but I wanted it enough so I kept at it and endured the pain. Amazingly, at about hour number seven, it seemed to get easier. Now that I am a licensed helicopter pilot with over one hundred hours, it seems almost brainless. But I had to endure a lot of discomfort for my subconscious mind to receive adequate programming. My subconscious mind learned the requirements of flying a helicopter to the point that my conscious mind could be freed to concentrate on other things. I was in the zone.

You are going to be in the zone. You are going to program your subconscious mind to the point that you are successful in making good exercise and nutrition choices every day.

Have you ever willed yourself to change and found that it just didn't work?

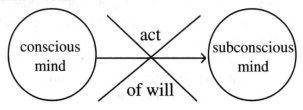

The Human Mind

How is it that we cannot have the willpower to do those positive things we desire? An understanding of the human mind will answer that question.

Our minds work in at least two dimensions. The conscious mind with which you are reading this material is the part of your mind that you are aware of. It is very limited in its capacity for storage or thought. It makes very few of our daily decisions. Our subconscious minds have extraordinary capacity for storage and thought and make the vast majority of our decisions.

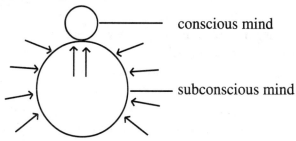

conscious mind

subconscious mind

Our minds were made this way for a reason. There is so much information to process that our subconscious mind has to play an active role. For example, if you are standing at a DO NOT WALK sign at a busy intersection, your conscious mind is aware of the sign telling you to wait. Your subconscious mind is aware of the people around you, and it is keeping you at a culturally appropriate distance from others while monitoring the traffic to maintain your safety. It is calculating the speed of the passing vehicles to verify that they will stop prior to your stepping in front of them. It is recording the color and style of the clothing and gender of other bystanders while at the same time monitoring your heart and breathing rates and managing your balance and muscle movement as you begin to walk.

The tremendous amount of data that must be processed requires a huge storage area that can make thousands of daily decisions automatically. **We become creatures of habit due**

to necessity.

You cannot order a computer to process information in a certain way. You must program the computer.

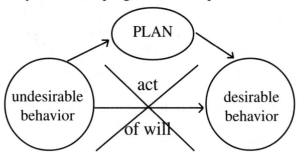

We are different from all other creatures in that we can choose to change our behaviors. This choice is made in the conscious mind. Most of it, however, is carried out through the subconscious mind via habits.

I'm not an animal!
— The Elephant Man

Priorities

You might remember from high school psychology class that Maslow suggested we have a hierarchy of needs. He believed we are driven to fulfill these needs beginning with the biological level. Survival is our strongest drive.

Self-Actualization
Needs to fulfill potential, have meaningful goals

Esteem
Needs for confidence, sense of worth and competence, self-esteem and respect of others

Attachment
Needs to belong, to affiliate, to love and be loved

Safety
Needs for security, comfort, tranquility, freedom from fear

Biological
Needs for food, water, oxygen, rest, sexual expression, release from tension

Our subconscious minds prioritize for security and survival. We are driven to eat due to an instinct for survival. We conserve energy and avoid exercise because of the instinct for survival. To make matters worse, our rational mind, which controls our need for personal achievement, is instinctually less of a priority for our subconscious minds. But we are human and we can choose our own priorities. Every great thing in our lives comes from our capacity to choose.

It may seem that the subconscious mind is a barrier to your goals. On the contrary, it is your greatest asset if you understand the process.

Habits

Do you know that it takes about a month to acquire a bad habit? If you ever were a smoker, you may remember your first cigarette. Chances are you weren't a natural born smoker. You hacked and coughed your way through those first few packs and probably even experienced some nausea. But you wanted to fit in and you wanted to be like the people around you. You programmed yourself to become a smoker.

There are several things to note here. First, you had a goal. Second, you found that it was difficult and required discomfort and perseverance. Third, it required an environment for change. You had a support group of smoking friends, who kept you at the desired task if you wavered. If you were determined, you probably acquired the habit of smoking in about thirty days.

The habits of exercise and eating well are also acquired along the same lines. You set attainable short-term goals. You endure the moderate discomfort and inconvenience. You create an environment for change that includes friends who share the same goals. When you miss a day or cheat on your diet, you get back on schedule and continue. You will find that about thirty days of persistence will produce the desired habits.

Let's dig a little deeper into how our mind either supports or sabotages our intentions. In addition to prioritizing for survival and comfort, our subconscious mind forms a self-concept from a very early age. As children, we got thousands of messages that shaped our self-concept. These messages come to us when we are vulnerable, clumsy and needy, so we accept much of this information as valid without rational consideration. We make up scripts in which we live out our lives, and we seek out roles that are comfortable rather than finding what might be best for us.

Most everyone's childhood included some adults who were not kind and nurturing and some children who were cruel. If you were exposed to people who were harsh and uncaring, it is possible you received some programming that has diminished your sense of self-worth.

Self-labels

We label ourselves based on these early recordings and then we make many of our decisions based on often erroneous information. Phil McGraw says it well in *Self Matters*. He believes that ten defining moments, seven critical choices and five influential people form our self-concept. I believe he is accurate. It is amazing that we would live out our lives based on such nominal and often inaccurate notions and childhood experiences

If we understand the role and power of the subconscious mind, we can make it work for us. Very few of our daily decisions are made by the conscious mind, so we must create an environment for change if we want to change behaviors.

We often engage in behaviors that are not rational or helpful, and we do this because there is some payoff. A wife might pick a fight with her husband so he will say bad things to her, which reaffirms her poor self-esteem. A man might cheat on his diet because he feels he doesn't deserve to be healthy.

Remember, we first seek comfort rather than those things that might be best for us.

Can you make a list of ten things you may do that are comfortable for you, but not best for you?

Self-talk

We engage in self-dialogue on a continual basis. As you are reading this, you stop momentarily and discuss the ideas with yourself. You might wander off and talk about other things as well. Self-talk is an extremely influential factor in our lives. What do you say to yourself when you look into the mirror? Chances are you're probably very hard on yourself. Self-talk is a habit, a habit that can be changed.

Men seem to have fewer problems with this issue. They're generally able to stand in front of the mirror with their gut hanging down, do a double biceps pose, and tell themselves how great they look. You may know one of these men.

Women need to work on self-talk that is helpful and accurate. Through the rest of this chapter, I am going to highlight helpful self-talk. Try to remember some of it and put it into practice.

When you were a bit younger, you might remember Stuart Smalley on Saturday Night Live. His daily affirmation was, "I'm smart enough, I'm good enough, and doggone it, people like me." Maybe that's over the top, but it's a lot better than, "I can't stick with a diet or I'm too lazy to exercise" or "my butt is too big."

Self-talk that is helpful and accurate will reinforce the labels and life scripts you choose. I'm a helicopter pilot today because I chose to be. When I was humiliated and tempted to quit, I told myself I could do it. I kept telling myself I could do it until I could do it.

You need to start telling yourself that you can exercise and eat right. Your life depends on it.

Environment

People become like those who surround them. One of the great advantages of being a Curves member is the supportive environment. The camaraderie of other women who share your goals and desires is a great asset. You are going to see women in much worse shape than you who are moving around the circuit, sweating and working and achieving. Their example will inspire you.

There will be people working there that are interested in you. They will teach you what you need to know about exercise and nutrition. Your weight and measurements will be taken and goals will be set. Each month you will be weighed and measured so you can see your progress.

Tell everyone what you are doing - shout it from the rooftops. This will increase your motivation and accountability, and enlist the help of those who care about you.

What kind of images do you expose yourself to every day? I am in the habit of getting up a half hour before everyone else. I take that time to casually plan my day. I pray quietly and cover people and circumstances. I read something inspirational, and I read my bible for a few minutes. I do this every day because it sets the day in motion calmly and deliberately.

During the day, I don't have music or TV on all the time. I take time to think about things without distractions. When I do listen to the radio, I choose uplifting music or information. Soap operas may be an escape, but at what price? They may expose you to a value system you don't want to get comfortable with.

Romance novels could be replaced with something equally entertaining but far more constructive. Your choices about how you use your time are important because you literally become what you are exposed to. Creating an environment for success requires a thousand deliberate choices made and remade every day.

Attitude

Before we get to the plan, let's talk about this thing called attitude. I define ATTITUDE as that state of mind through which you filter all information and make all decisions.

Those who have a sorry attitude about life generally have a sorry life. Our basic attitude is probably due to a series of events that we had no control over or a few people who treated us poorly. But we can choose our own attitude and determine our own quality of life. In fact, attitudes can be consciously built, and they must be nurtured and protected.

Chuck Swindoll says that attitude is a more significant factor in determining success in life than aptitude, opportunity, luck and all three combined.

Attitude is a product of your character, self-labeling, self-talk, habits and environment. As we've discussed, these are all products of choices you have made or choices you can make.

The character choices that will influence attitude come from the confidence of deferring gratification and enduring the pain of change and growth. You become stronger, smarter and more confident as you experience success. The habits you acquire will either build up or break down a positive mental attitude.

Self-labeling can be modified as you reassess who you really are. You can actively choose your self-concept and live the life of significance you were destined for.

Helpful and accurate self-talk will reassure you of your value and purpose on a moment-to-moment basis.

The environment you create and maintain for yourself will reinforce this mind through which you filter all information and make all decisions.

Goals

You should now consider those specific behavioral changes you would like to accomplish. You are not likely to end up where you want to be if you don't know where you are going.

Specific and Written

Goals should be clear and achievable. You must write them down and refer to them regularly, so place them on a refrigerator door or your vanity mirror. As you accomplish goals, cross them off. As your goals become good new habits, set new goals. Always be aware of your destination.

Society has perpetrated a cruel hoax on women in America. Images of women with unattainable and unhealthy bodies cover our magazines and movie screens. Free yourself from these unrealistic demands. You probably cannot look like them and it would be unhealthy if you did.

Self-talk

I'm not going to end up where I want to be if I don't know where I'm going.

Motivation

Set goals that will be motivating as well as reasonable. If you need to lose a hundred pounds, don't shoot for ten pounds. Go for fifty and your life will change in positive ways.

Exercise, nutrition and weight-loss goals should be tied to something motivating. Holidays with friends and family, reunions, and vacations all provide a deadline that will motivate you to defer gratification. Picture yourself on the beach wearing a bathing suit and feeling comfortable. A longer-term goal may involve attending a grandchild's graduation or wedding. Pictures that portray these events should be placed around your home and office to continually remind you of why you must endure the discomfort of change.

Enjoy the Journey

Great things take time. They involve many small steps rather than a few large steps. If you have a hundred pounds to lose, it can be daunting. If you look at the mountain you wish to climb, it will overwhelm you, so look at the first step. An amazing thing happens with goals: when you've gone as far as you can see, you can see farther. With exercise and nutritional goals, even nominal efforts, will stop the downward spiral of poor health. With the Curves plan that protects muscle tissue as you lose body fat, each accomplishment is more likely to be retained. You will not immediately go back to where you were, as you might have in the past. If you lose twenty pounds of the one hundred you would like to lose, falling off the wagon for a few weeks will only take you back a short distance. Two steps forward and one step backward will still get you to your destination. Enjoy the journey - it will ultimately be the best part.

Obstacles

Any great achievement will have obstacles. As a pilot, I get in my airplane and head off in a certain direction. If I encounter an area of bad weather, I turn around and come back home, right? Wrong! I simply change direction, go around the weather and get back on course. I may not get where I intended to go as quickly and efficiently as I had intended, but I get there anyway. As you encounter lapses on your diet, don't be overwhelmed by failure. Any significant achievement will have times of failure, so just get back on course. You may not arrive as quickly and efficiently as you desire, but you will arrive.

Confusing Disappointment with Disaster

I have a friend who would like to quit smoking. At age forty, he had a cancerous lesion removed from his arm. I like to remind him that it was his smoking arm. He has a nine-year-old son who has asthma. There is lots of motivation here, yet he continually fails in his goal to stop smoking. He likes to say he's not a quitter. He always starts off well. He goes several weeks without a single cigarette. He endures the discomfort of tobacco withdrawal and at about the three week point finds himself in a moment of weakness. He smokes one cigarette. He is so overwhelmed with failure that he immediately becomes a pack-a-day smoker again. Rather than moving forward around the obstacle, he gives up completely. He confuses a minor disappointment with disaster. Achieving any significant goal will have disappointments.

Be Your Own Best Friend

I'm not a cynical person, but I realize that other people can be selfish and insensitive to my needs. Don't wait for others to encourage and motivate you to value yourself – do it yourself. I have found that about eighty-percent of people really don't care what happens to me, and most of the other twenty-percent are actually glad when bad things happen.

"I'm a Mog, half man and half dog.
I'm my own best friend."
— John Candy in the movie Spaceballs

There are probably very few people who have risen above their own survival needs and have time to care for you, so take care of yourself. If you want to be around for others then you must take care of yourself. There is no better care that you can give your children than the example of living well.

Steps in the Right Direction

Let's make a list of ten easy changes you would like to make in each of three areas of your life. I'll start with five and you fill in five. After you thoughtfully complete these lists, post them where you will see them during the day. After a few weeks of effort, you will find that these behaviors occur naturally. They will become habits. You will then be ready to make a new list of a few larger goals.

ACTIVITY GOALS

1. Walk ten minutes daily.
2. Take the stairs.
3. "Run" errands rather than drive them.
4. Do 10 sit-ups and 10 push-ups each morning.
5. Go to Curves 3 times this week.
6. _____
7. _____
8. _____
9. _____
10. _____

NUTRITIONAL GOALS

1. Switch to diet drinks (later to tea and water).
2. Eat 25 grams of fiber daily.
3. Eat 2 servings of fruit and 3 servings of vegetables daily.
4. Drink water at least 4 times daily.
5. Leave food on your plate.
6. _____
7. _____
8. _____
9. _____
10. _____

MENTAL GOALS

1. Stop watching Jerry Springer and soap operas.

2. Read something inspirational daily.

3. When asked how you are, answer "Great!"

4. Look in the mirror each day and find something positive about your appearance.

5. Pray each morning.

6. _____

7. _____

8. _____

9. _____

10. _____

Self-talk

I feel happy. I feel healthy. I feel terrific!

The Greatest Power

I would be remiss if I didn't share with you the greatest power for change and self-worth. As a born-again Christian, I have come to personally know God. He spoke the world into existence and holds every atom in check. He created you and me and gave us the choice of free will. When our forefather chose poorly, God loved us enough to redeem us and make a way for relationship once again.

When you come to know who God really is and how much He loves you, there is no greater affirmation of your value. There is no greater potential for power and significance. You can do all things through Christ who strengthens you. You can become a person with great self-control, joy and purpose.

Chapter Review

*Learn from past failures rather than repeat them.

*A rational plan for change is more reliable than an emotional foundation.

*Changing behavior requires the support of the subconscious mind.

*People have the ability to choose the way they live. Habits, self-labels, self-talk and environment may be chosen to support a better quality of life.

*Attitude is that state of mind through which you filter all information and make all decisions.

*Goals must be realistic, exciting and written.

CHAPTER XI

THE CURVES
WEIGHT-LOSS METHOD

- **Preview Of The Program**

- **Practical Considerations**

- **Getting Started**

- **Weight Chart**

- **Exercise Chart**

- **Measurement Chart**

- **Phase I, Shopping List & Meal Plans**

- **Phase II & Meal Plans**

- **Phase III**

- **Chapter Review**

Our method for permanent weight-loss is divided into three phases which are explained below.

Phase I goals:

Learn how to lose weight

Get off to a great start

Acquire the tools and the confidence to control your weight

Phase II goals:

Continue losing safely until you either reach your goal or hit a plateau

Phase III goals

Raise metabolism so you do not have to diet forever to maintain your weight-loss

or

Raise metabolism so you can start losing weight again, until you reach your goal

Preview of the Program

Phase I

Phase I is the strictest part of the plan. You will choose the most advantageous method of dieting for you, based on the tests in Chapter V. If the tests show you are carbohydrate intolerant, you may enjoy the advantage of a higher protein and lower carbohydrate plan. The advantage of this plan is that you can eat more food and still lose weight. However, you must limit your carbohydrates to 20 grams per day (after subtractng free foods). If the tests show you are calorie sensitive, you must eat fewer calories, as well as limiting carbohydrates. The calorie sensitive plan calls for 1200 calories and 60 grams of carbohydrates per day (after subtracting free foods).

Phase I should produce significant weight-loss. Stay on

the stricter Phase I plan for one or two weeks depending on the amount of weight you need to lose. If you have less than twenty pounds to lose, one week is sufficient. If you have twenty or more pounds to lose, two weeks is appropriate.

It is very motivating to lose weight quickly. However, for periods longer than two weeks, you need wider variety and larger amounts of food than Phase I provides.

Phase I will allow you to acquire the skill and confidence to lose weight when you need to. This tool is an important part of Phase III.

Phase II

After one or two weeks on Phase I, you will move on to Phase II which has a larger amount and variety of food. If the higher protein advantages are working for you, you should continue following the carbohydrate intolerant plan; however, you may increase your daily grams of carbohydrates from 20 to 60 (after subtracting free foods). On the calorie sensitive plan, you may increase your caloric intake from 1200 to 1600 calories per day but keep your carbohydrate intake at 60 grams per day (after subtracting free foods).

Phase II will continue to produce weight-loss, but at a slower rate than Phase I. You should expect to lose two pounds per week initially and then slow to a pound per week as your metabolism lowers. When you reach your weight-loss goal or your weight-loss slows to less than one pound per week, you must move on to Phase III. You never want to stay on a diet when you have hit a plateau. You have hit a plateau because your metabolism has been lowered as a result of the accumulation of starvation hormones.

Phase III

The objective of Phase III is to raise your metabolism. Only with an adequate metabolic rate can you eat well and maintain your goal weight. You must realize that, after living on stored energy for a number of weeks, your metabolic rate has decreased. Starvation hormones have saturated your blood and have increased your energy efficiency. Your body has responded appropriately to a period of famine, just as it was designed to do.

Your objective is to eliminate the starvation hormones from your body. You must begin to eat so that your body will cease the production of these hormones. We recommend you eat an amount of calories that are healthy for your body size and level of activity. You will gain weight.

When you begin to eat normally after dieting, you will rehydrate. The first couple of pounds are water weight. After eating normally for several days, you will gain a couple of pounds of water and perhaps a pound of body fat.

Don't panic, you know exactly what to do. Go on the strict Phase I diet for two or three days. You will lose the water weight, and after two days or so, you will lose the pound of fat as well. Work with an ideal weight and a high weight of three to five pounds over that. If you are a large person, your water weight can easily fluctuate by five pounds.

Remember that eating raises metabolism and dieting produces starvation hormones that lower metabolism. You must eat to increase your metabolic rate and to stop the production of starvation hormones, and you will initially regain a small amount of weight. The key is to never regain more weight than you can lose in two or three days. That's how long your body can diet before it begins to produce starvation hormones. Eating adequately and allowing time to pass will dissipate the starvation hormones that have saturated your body following weeks of dieting.

Permanent results require that you be prepared to follow the Phase I diet for two or three days whenever you reach your high weight. Of course, you must weigh yourself every day to find out when you have reached your high weight. You will lose that small amount of weight (three pounds), and then return to normal eating until the next time you reach your high weight. Eventually most people find that they may eat normally for as many as twenty-nine days a month if they will diet for a few days whenever necessary.

Practical Considerations

Eating five or six small meals every day rather than two or three large ones has several advantages:

• You will not get hungry between meals, so you will be less apt to cheat.

• Your body expends a lot of energy as it gears up to digest those meals.

• Frequent stimulation of your thyroid gland throughout the day will keep your metabolic rate higher. The thyroid gland responds during digestion by producing T3 and T4 metabolic hormones.

There are free foods that may be consumed without regard to their calorie or carbohydrate content. You do not count their calorie or carbohydrate content due to the amount of roughage they contain. Many of their calories are not accessible during digestion. They include: green leafy vegetables, cabbage, celery, cucumbers, non-sweet onions, garlic, mushrooms, peppers, non-sweet pickles, radishes, summer squash and zucchini. Good flavoring choices are mustard and lemon juice.

One Curves shake per day is allowed as a free food, even though it contains 200 calories and 20 grams of carbohydrates. We have found that some people become constipated when they diet, and the herbal blend in our shake helps to keep things moving. We believe this benefit more than compensates for the extra calories. If you consume more than one shake in a day, you must count the calories and carbohydrates in any shake after the first one.

Planning is crucial to your success. Most people find it beneficial to begin their diet on a Monday. Be sure to take your grocery list with you to the store so that you have everything you need before your starting day. You should prepare snacks and meals in advance whenever possible. The Curves Diet Workbook is a great tool to help you stay with the diet for the entire 6 weeks. It contains daily food plans, recipes, journaling space, weekly lessons, and many references.

Learn to calculate portion sizes and purchase a food reference book. The palm of a woman's hand (the surface and thickness) is equivalent to 3 ounces of meat. Make a loose fist — the area from the wrist to the tip of the knuckles is about one cup of food. A good reference book is *The Encyclopedia of Food Values* by Corinne T. Netzer.

Each meal plan in this book has seven days of menus. Each day is labeled for a particular day of the week, but you are not limited to this schedule. You may choose any individual day that best fits your schedule. Perhaps you are not a breakfast eater. Monday, Wednesday or Friday may be the best plan for you. Having a large, late lunch today? Check out the Friday or Saturday plan. Sunday is perfect for breakfast before church followed by a leisurely lunch. Eating out is fun and this plan makes dining with friends a breeze. Any proteins may be exchanged for other proteins and vegetables for other similar vegetables.

Fruits are generally high in sugar. Fruit juices are even higher. Wise fruit choices will include cantaloupe, honeydew melons, and strawberries. Bananas, grapes, apples, oranges and watermelons are out for a while.

There is no doubt that artificial sweeteners are not good for you; however, you must choose your battles. If diet drinks or coffee and tea with artificial sweeteners will help you to stay on your diet, they are the lesser of evils. The same goes for diet Jello or other similar foods.

Getting Started

Have a Curves instructor weigh and measure you the morning you begin. Have your body fat percentage checked as well. Record this information on your measurement charts. Weighing in will be a weekly event. Measurement of inches and body fat will be done at the beginning, at week four, and at the end of the six-week program. You should weigh under similar conditions each week (before a meal, wearing similar clothing, at the same time of day). Write down your goals for weight-loss, inches loss, and ideal body fat percentage.

If you have any health concerns, be sure you visit with your doctor before starting this or any other diet. The advantages of a higher protein diet are not worth putting your health at risk. Be sure you are in good health before you choose the higher protein plan.

Be Sure To

Drink 8 glasses of water every day

Take a good multi-vitamin/mineral supplement

Eat, but don't cheat

Weight Chart

Write your beginning weight in the top box in the left column and enter one pound decreases down the column. Place an X in the corresponding weekly weight amounts. Place your goal weight in the goal box. This graph will help you to visualize your success.

Start   **Goal**

Week 1	Week 2	Week 3	Week 4	Week 5	Week 6	Week 7	
185							
184							
183							
182	X						
181							
180		X					

Start   **Goal**

Week 1	Week 2	Week 3	Week 4	Week 5	Week 6	Week 7	

Exercise Chart

Keep a record of weekly exercise. Each day place an X in the box for each ten minutes of exercise performed. Write the type of exercise and how much energy you felt afterward, 1-5 with 5 the highest.

Week #	Day or Date	Minutes per day Each box = 10 min.								Type of Exercise	Post Exercise Energy level 1-5 (most)
1											
2											
3											
4											
5											
6											

Measurement Chart

Beginning	Week 4	Final	Goal
MEASUREMENTS	**MEASUREMENTS**	**MEASUREMENTS**	**MEASUREMENTS**
Bust _____	Bust _____	Bust _____	Bust _____
Waist _____	Waist _____	Waist _____	Waist _____
Abdomen _____	Abdomen _____	Abdomen _____	Abdomen _____
Hips _____	Hips _____	Hips _____	Hips _____
Thighs _____	Thighs _____	Thighs _____	Thighs _____
Calves _____	Calves _____	Calves _____	Calves _____
Arms _____	Arms _____	Arms _____	Arms _____
Weight _____	Weight _____	Weight _____	Weight _____
Body Fat % _____	Body Fat % _____	Body Fat % _____	Body Fat % _____
Fat lbs. _____	Fat lbs. _____	Fat lbs. _____	Fat lbs. _____
Date _____	Date _____	Date _____	Date _____

Phase I Meal Plans

Phase I is the strictest phase of the diet, but also the shortest. You should have taken the tests in Chapter V to determine whether you are carbohydrate intolerant or calorie sensitive. If you are carbohydrate intolerant, you may enjoy the advantage of the higher protein plan, which means you can eat more food and still lose weight. Otherwise you should follow the calorie restricted plan. If you are one of the 25% who seem to be both carbohydrate and calorie sensitive, you may start with the higher protein plan. If you haven't lost any weight within a few days, go to the calorie plan, or if your weight-loss stops following several weeks of success with the higher protein plan, move to the calorie plan.

The higher protein plan allows you to consume all of the meat, cheeses, eggs, seafood and poultry that you desire. You must keep your carbohydrate intake at or below 20 grams per day (after subtracting free foods). Try to eat lean meats that are broiled or baked, never fried. Keep fat consumption at a moderate level.

The calorie version allows 1200 calories daily. About 40% of these calories should be from protein. You must not eat more than 60 grams of carbohydrates (after subtracting free foods) during Phase I. This will allow your body to feed your muscles while accessing stored fat for energy.

If you have more than twenty pounds to lose, remain on Phase I for two weeks. Those who have less to lose may move on to Phase II after one week.

Enjoy your free foods and the variety they provide. One Curves shake per day (made with skim milk) will give you a moment of pleasure by providing a treat.

Your weight-loss goal for the first week will be from 4 to 6 pounds. The second week, you should lose 3 pounds. The difference is that you will lose a larger amount of water weight during the first few days. The scale is only one measurement device. It reflects many factors and may not be an accurate measure of progress. Inches and body fat will be measured soon but pay attention to how your clothes feel as the days go by.

SHOPPING LIST

VEGETABLES
Artichoke Hearts, Seabrook frozen
Asparagus
Broccoli
Carrots
Cauliflower
Celery
Cucumber
Green Beans
Lettuce
Mushrooms
Okra
Okra Gumbo
Onion
Spinach
Tomato
Zucchini

_____
_____
_____
_____
_____
_____

DAIRY
Cheese — grated
Cheese — Havarti
Cheese — Mozzarella
Cheese — Parmesan
Cheese — White American
Cottage cheese, small curd
Eggs
Milk — skim
Yogurt, plain, whole milk

_____
_____
_____
_____
_____
_____

FRUIT
Blueberries
Cantaloupe
Honeydew Melon
Raspberries
Strawberries

_____
_____
_____
_____

MEAT
Chicken, fajita
Chicken, grilled breast
Hamburger
Pork Chop, center cut, lean
Rainbow Trout
Roast Beef, shaved
Salmon
Sirloin Steak
Steakburger, lean meat only
Tuna Salad
Tunafish, in water
Turkey Breast
Turkey Ham, cold cuts
Turkey Sausage
Turkey, patty — breakfast

_____
_____
_____
_____

CALORIE VERSION ONLY
Melba Toast
Oatmeal Bread —
   Pepperidge Farms 'Very Thin'

PHASE II ONLY
Potato
Rice — long grain wild

Curves Weight–loss Plan Phase I

Meal	1200cal	High Protein/20g. Carbs
Meal 1	shake	shake
Meal 2	1/2 C cottage cheese 1/2 C strawberries	cottage cheese strawberries
Meal 3	4 oz lean steakburger (meat only) salad	lean steakburger (meat only) salad
Meal 4	3 pieces Melba toast 3 oz tuna salad	tuna salad pickles
Meal 5	4 oz turkey breast broiled or grilled 1 oz Parmesan stir fry mixture- onions, mushrooms, spinach	turkey breast broiled or grilled any cheese stir fry mixture- onions, mushrooms, spinach
Meal 6	6 slices turkey ham (no Carbs)	sliced turkey ham & cheese

WATER — 8, 7, 6, 5, 4, 3, 2, 1

Meal	1200cal	High Protein/20g. Carbs
Meal 1	1 large soft boiled egg 1 small tomato sliced	eggs any style 1 small tomato sliced
Meal 2	1/2 C cubed cantaloupe 1/2 C cottage cheese	cottage cheese 1/2 C cubed cantaloupe
Meal 3	4 oz fajita chicken strips Salad	fajita chicken strips shredded cheese salad
Meal 4	shake	shake
Meal 5	4 oz broiled sirloin broccoli cauliflower salad	broiled sirloin cabbage
Meal 6	3 cubes of cheese	cheese pickles

WATER — 8, 7, 6, 5, 4, 3, 2, 1

CURVES WEIGHT-LOSS PLAN PHASE I

Meal	1200cal	High Protein/20g. Carbs
Meal 1	8 oz plain yogurt & 1/4 C blueberries blended together	plain yogurt & 1/4 C blueberries blended together
Meal 2	shake	shake
Meal 3	chef salad — salad 1 oz grated cheese 4 oz roast beef	chef salad — grated cheese shaved turkey, beef & ham
Meal 4	3 pieces Melba toast 3 oz tuna salad	tuna salad cheese pickles
Meal 5	7 oz broiled salmon zucchini	broiled salmon zucchini
Meal 6	3 slices turkey ham (no Carbs)	turkey ham (no Carbs)

WATER — 8, 7, 6, 5, 4, 3, 2, 1

Meal	1200cal	High Protein/20g. Carbs
Meal 1	1 large poached egg 2 turkey sausage links 1 piece 'Very Thin' Pepperidge Farm oatmeal toast	eggs & sausage
Meal 2	1/2 C cottage cheese 1/2 C baby carrots - raw	cottage cheese
Meal 3	6 oz tuna packed in water salad	tuna packed in water pickles
Meal 4	shake	shake
Meal 5	4 oz. grilled chicken breast mushrooms onions 3 oz Seabrook artichoke hearts asparagus	grilled chicken breast cheese celery with cream cheese
Meal 6		cold cuts

WATER — 8, 7, 6, 5, 4, 3, 2, 1

Meal	1200cal	High Protein/20g. Carbs
Meal 1	8 oz plain yogurt & 1/4 C strawberries	eggs & bacon
Meal 2	1/2 C cottage cheese 1/2 C cantaloupe	cottage cheese celery & peanut butter
Meal 3	4 oz broiled center cut lean pork chop salad zucchini	broiled center cut lean pork chop salad zucchini
Meal 4		
Meal 5	shake	shake
Meal 6	4 oz egg & tuna salad 3 cubes cheese celery	egg & tuna salad cheese celery

WATER — 8, 7, 6, 5, 4, 3, 2, 1

Meal	1200cal	High Protein/20g. Carbs
Meal 1	1 slice oatmeal bread 1 slice tomato 1 slice Havarti cheese 2 turkey patties	eggs 1 small tomato cheese
Meal 2	shake	shake
Meal 3	1/4 lb hamburger patties salad	hamburger patties cheese
Meal 4		
Meal 5	4 oz rainbow trout 1 C okra gumbo salad	4 oz rainbow trout okra gumbo salad
Meal 6	4 oz yogurt blended with 1/2 C raspberries	cold cuts cheese pickles

WATER — 8, 7, 6, 5, 4, 3, 2, 1

Meal	1200cal	High Protein/20g. Carbs
Meal 1	2 large eggs over easy 3 sausage links 1 tomato — sliced	eggs over easy sausage links 1 tomato — sliced
Meal 2		
Meal 3	4 oz grilled chicken breast 1/2 C green beans salad	grilled chicken breast cheese 1/2 C green beans
Meal 4	1 C cottage cheese 1 wedge honeydew melon	cottage cheese celery
Meal 5	1/4 lb grilled or broiled shrimp spinach cauliflower	grilled or broiled shrimp spinach cauliflower
Meal 6	shake	shake

WATER — 8, 7, 6, 5, 4, 3, 2, 1

Phase II Meal Plans

You should have successfully completed the strict Phase I plan. It gets much easier from here. It is important that you increase the quantity and variety of your foods.

The higher protein plan continues to allow the unlimited consumption of protein foods such as meat, cheeses, eggs, seafood and poultry. You may now increase your daily grams of carbohydrates from 20 to 60 (after subtracting free foods). Be sure to enjoy the variety of free foods that are available to you.

The calorie plan allows an increase from 1200 to 1600 calories daily while keeping your carbohydrates at or under 60 grams (after subtracting free foods). You should still consume about 40% of these calories as protein.

Your weekly weight-loss goal during Phase II is from 1 to 3 pounds. You will lose weight more slowly during Phase II because you are eating more and because your metabolism is beginning to slow. As you burn stored energy (body fat), your body begins to produce starvation hormones. After an extended period of time, enough starvation hormones will have been produced to lower your metabolism to levels that do not allow for continued weight-loss.

If your daily metabolic rate was 3000 calories at the beginning of Phase I, it may have been lowered to 2600 by now. This is still high enough to continue losing weight. Consuming 1600 calories per day creates a 1000-calorie daily deficit that would result in a one-pound loss of body fat every three and a half days, because each pound of fat contains 3500 calories. As long as your metabolism is sufficiently high, you will continue to lose weight while staying on Phase II.

You will go off of Phase II when you stop losing weight or you reach your goal. There are six weeks of measurement records included in this book. If you are still losing weight, stay on Phase II as long as you can. If you reach your goal prior to the end of the six weeks, move on to Phase III.

Meal	1600cal	High Protein/60g. Carbs
Meal 1	shake	shake
Meal 2	1/2 C cottage cheese 1/2 C strawberries	cottage cheese 1/2 C strawberries

Meal 3	8 oz lean
	  steakburger
	  (meat only)
		lean
		  steakburger
		  (meat only)

Meal 4	3 pieces Melba toast 5 oz tuna salad	3 pieces Melba toast tuna salad dill or sour pickles

Meal 5	4 oz turkey breast
	  broiled or grilled
	1 oz parmesan cheese
	stir fry onions,
	  mushrooms, &
	  spinach
	1/2 C wild rice
		turkey breast
		  broiled or grilled
		cheese
		stir fry onions,
		  mushrooms, &
		  spinach

Meal 6	6 slices turkey ham (no Carbs)	cold cuts & cheese any raw vegetables

WATER — 8, 7, 6, 5, 4, 3, 2, 1

Meal	1600cal	High Protein/60g. Carbs
Meal 1	1 large soft boiled egg 1 tomato sliced	soft boiled eggs 1 tomato sliced
Meal 2	1/2 C cubed cantaloupe 1/2 C cottage cheese	1/2 C cubed cantaloupe cottage cheese
Meal 3	6 oz fajita chicken strips 1 oz shredded cheese salad	fajita chicken strips shredded cheese salad
Meal 4	shake	shake
Meal 5	6 oz broiled sirloin broccoli cauliflower salad	broiled sirloin broccoli cauliflower salad
Meal 6	3 cubes of cheese	cold cuts & cheese

WATER — 8, 7, 6, 5, 4, 3, 2, 1

Meal	1600cal	High Protein/60g. Carbs
Meal 1	8 oz plain yogurt & 1/4 C blueberries blended together	8 oz plain yogurt & 1/4 C blueberries blended together
Meal 2	shake	shake
Meal 3	salad 1 oz grated cheese 4 oz shaved roast beef	salad grated cheese shaved roast beef
Meal 4	3 pieces Melba toast 6 oz tuna salad	3 pieces Melba toast tuna salad
Meal 5	8 oz broiled salmon zucchini 1/2 C wild rice	broiled salmon zucchini
Meal 6	6 slices turkey ham (no Carbs)	cold cuts & cheese any raw vegetables

WATER — 8, 7, 6, 5, 4, 3, 2, 1

Meal	1600cal	High Protein/60g. Carbs

Meal 1	1 large poached egg
	2 links turkey sausage
	1 piece 'Very Thin'
	  Pepperidge Farm
	  oatmeal toast
		1 large poached egg
		2 links turkey sausage

Meal 2	1/2 C cottage cheese 1/2 C baby carrots	cottage cheese 1/2 C baby carrots

Meal 3	6.3 oz tuna,
	  packed in water
	salad
	4 cubes cheese
		tuna,
		  packed in water
		salad
		cheese

Meal 4	shake	shake

Meal 5	4 oz grilled chicken
	  breast
	1 oz grated cheese
	mushrooms
	onions
	3 oz Seabrook
	  artichoke hearts
	asparagus
		grilled chicken
		  breast
		grated cheese
		mushrooms
		onions
		3 oz Seabrook
		  artichoke hearts
		asparagus

Meal 6		

WATER — 8, 7, 6, 5, 4, 3, 2, 1

CURVES WEIGHT-LOSS PLAN PHASE II
FRIDAY

Meal	1600cal	High Protein/60g. Carbs
Meal 1	8 oz plain yogurt & 1/4 C sliced strawberries	plain yogurt & 1/4 C sliced strawberries
Meal 2	1/2 C cottage cheese 1/2 C cantaloupe 6 pieces turkey ham	cottage cheese 1/2 C cantaloupe turkey ham
Meal 3	4 oz broiled center cut pork chops salad zucchini 2 potato skins with Parmesan	broiled center cut pork chops salad zucchini
Meal 4		
Meal 5	shake	shake
Meal 6	4 oz egg & tuna salad 3 cubes cheese celery	egg & tuna salad cheese celery

WATER — 8, 7, 6, 5, 4, 3, 2, 1

Meal	1600cal	High Protein/60g. Carbs
Meal 1	1 slice oatmeal toast 1 tomato sliced 1 slice cheese 2 turkey patties	1 slice oatmeal toast 1 tomato sliced cheese turkey patties
Meal 2	shake	shake

Meal 3	1/2 lb grilled
	  hamburger meat
	salad
	1 slice cheese
		grilled hamburger
		  meat
		salad
		cheese

Meal 4		
Meal 5	8 oz rainbow trout 1 C okra gumbo salad	rainbow trout okra gumbo salad
Meal 6	1/2 C raspberries 4 oz yogurt	1/2 C raspberries yogurt cold cuts cheese

WATER — 8, 7, 6, 5, 4, 3, 2, 1

Meal	1600cal	High Protein/60g. Carbs
Meal 1	2 large eggs over easy 3 sausage links 1 tomato — sliced	eggs over easy sausage links 1 tomato — sliced
Meal 2		

Meal 3	4 oz grilled chicken
	  breast
	1 oz mozzarella
	1/2 C green beans
	salad
	1/2 C wild rice
		grilled chicken
		  breast
		mozzarella
		1/2 C green beans
		salad

Meal 4	1 C cottage cheese
	1" wedge honeydew
	  melon
		cottage cheese
		1" wedge honeydew
		  melon

Meal 5	1/2 lb grilled or broiled
	  shrimp
	spinach
	cauliflower
		grilled or broiled
		  shrimp
		spinach
		cauliflower

Meal 6	shake	shake

WATER — 8, 7, 6, 5, 4, 3, 2, 1

Curves Weight-loss Plan

Day _____

Meal	1200cal / 1600cal	High Protein 20 g carbs/60g carbs
Meal 1		
Meal 2		
Meal 3		
Meal 4		
Meal 5		
Meal 6		

WATER — 8, 7, 6, 5, 4, 3, 2, 1

CURVES WEIGHT-LOSS PLAN

DAY_____

Meal	1200cal / 1600cal	High Protein 20 g carbs/60g carbs
Meal 1		
Meal 2		
Meal 3		
Meal 4		
Meal 5		
Meal 6		

WATER — 8, 7, 6, 5, 4, 3, 2, 1

Phase III

The objective of Phase III is to raise metabolism back to pre-diet levels. Phase III is not really a diet; in fact, it is mostly eating. Eating is what stops the production of starvation hormones and raises metabolism.

Other weight-loss programs would require you to continue dieting. A maintenance diet would have you perpetually diet, although at a slightly higher caloric intake, because they realize your metabolism will have diminished due to weeks of dieting. If your metabolism had been lowered to 2000 calories or less per day, they would have you consume no more than 2000 calories daily indefinitely. This perpetual dieting would perpetually lower your metabolism. These conventional methods probably contributed to your past failures.

Our Phase III plan requires that you go off of your diet when you either reach your goal or you hit a plateau. You must begin to eat to raise metabolism.

Because your metabolic rate decreased due to dieting, you will gain weight from eating more calories than you are burning. The key is to not gain more weight than you can lose in a 72-hour window (three days), because that's the amount of time it takes your body to begin producing starvation hormones.

The first couple of pounds that you immediately gain after going off a diet are water weight. Because you no longer need to access stored energy (body fat), your body will rehydrate. Establish a low weight and a high weight of three to five pounds over that. For example, you may want to weigh between 147 and 150 pounds. Lose down to 147 and begin to eat normally. Weigh yourself every day. You will probably gain a couple of pounds the first day or two. When the scale says 150, you will need to diet, but only for two or three days. The three pounds you gain probably represent two pounds of water and one pound of body fat.

Two or three days of dieting, (strict Phase I), will cause you to dehydrate and lose a couple of pounds of water and burn off the small amount of fat you gained. However, two or three days of dieting are not long enough to restimulate the production of starvation hormones. During this time, the starvation hormones that have saturated your body chemistry are dissipating. Eating and time will allow your metabolic rate to return to pre-diet levels. You must be sure to eat an adequate amount of food for your body size and activity level in order to increase metabolic rate, and you must never regain more weight than you can lose in a few days.

Your goal is to be able to eat normally for 29 days a month while having to diet for two or three days. Remember, outside the extreme of pregnancy, you probably gained weight at a rate of a half pound or so per month which became six pounds a year and thirty pounds after five years.

The following chart will help you to understand Phase III. Fill in your ideal weight and high weight. As you begin to start eating again, you will find that it takes longer and longer for you to regain those few pounds. Your prevailing metabolism is increasing as those starvation hormones are dissipating.

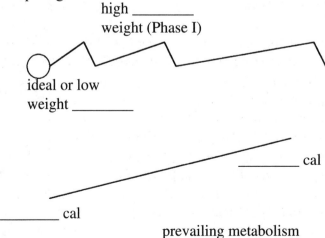

prevailing metabolism

More To Go

If you have hit a plateau prior to reaching your goal, you need to enjoy Phase III for a month or so. This will be time to eat abundantly and healthfully. You will be raising your metabolic rate back to pre-diet levels without regaining the weight you lost. When your metabolism is sufficiently high, you may begin the program with one or two weeks on Phase I and continue with Phase II. You will know when your metabolism is sufficiently high because you can eat several thousand calories daily and not gain weight. It may be necessary to cycle through the phases several times. It is comforting to know that at each cycle the weight need never be regained.

Low Metabolism

If you have been yo-yo dieting or have been dieting perpetually, you may have sabotaged your metabolism. You should disregard Phases I and II and begin with Phase III in order to raise metabolism. The process is the same. Your current weight will be your low or ideal weight and you should select a high weight that is a few pounds higher. Begin to eat at a caloric level that is high enough to raise your metabolism. Never gain more than a few pounds, then lose them by using the Phase I diet for two or three days. As your prevailing metabolism is raised, you should be able to eat normally for longer periods of time before you reach your high weight and must diet again.

When your metabolism is sufficiently high to start losing weight, you may follow the normal program, beginning with Phase I.

Everyone's biochemistry is a bit different. We have found that most people have great success with our methods. Be sure to set reasonable goals and continue to move forward. A few pounds less body fat and a few minutes more endurance will eventually take you where you want to be. Hopefully, you have found that this method of exercise and weight-loss has proven successful. See you at Curves!

Chapter Review

*Our approach to weight-loss utilizes three phases.

*Exercise and weight-loss charts help with account-ability and visualization of results.

*Phase I is the stricter of the phases.

*Phase II is the moderate phase.

*Phase III is not really a diet. It is a time to eat and raise metabolic rate.

*People who have sabotaged their metabolism may utilize Phase III to increase their metabolic rate.

Epilogue

People often ask me how, as a man, I became so committed to improving the quality of women's lives. It was less than seven years ago, at age forty, that I even realized myself.

One awful morning over thirty years ago, I was awakened by the passing schoolbus.

At age thirteen, my younger brothers and I were at home with our mother, Doris Joy Heavin. She had just passed her fortieth birthday. She was a committed mother of five children and had wrestled with emotional and physical problems most of her life. Her doctors had placed her on an array of medications with little benefit.

My younger brother, Paul, came into our room and told me that I'd better come because mother was sick. As I knelt beside her bed, I could feel the absence of warmth. I put my arms around her, first to feel for a sign of life, and then as a final embrace.

I took my younger brothers, ages eight and nine, in my arms and gently told them that our mother was in heaven.

Her premature death was unnecessary. The high blood pressure that contributed to the blood clot that took her life was unnecessary. Rather than medicate the symptoms, she could have dealt with the cause of her high blood pressure. We now know that exercise and proper nutrition will almost always alleviate the causes of hypertension and most other chronic diseases.

I finally understood the passion of my life as I stood before a group of a hundred women and realized I was subconsciously scanning the crowd for a glimpse of my mother.

It is my desire that no little boy has to find his mother as I found mine.

End Notes

1. Patricia Long, "Winning at Losing Weight," *Health* 10 (1, January-February 1996):64.

2. Califano, *Lose Weight for Life*, p. 56.

3. "Aging Boomers Lose the Battle of the Bulge," *USA Today*, (2, Jan. 1996) D2.

4. Wayne Campbell et al., Penn State University, study on exercise and aging, 1997.

5. "Rating the Diets," *Consumer Reports* 58 (6, June 93):354.

6. "Rockefeller Study" *NEJM*, (9 Mar. 95).

7. Claire M. Cassidy, *U. of Maryland & The Smithsonian Inst. Study* (1980).

8. Peter Brown, ed. *An Anthropological Perspective on Obesity from "Understanding and Applying Medical Anthropology"* edited by Peter Brown (1998).

9. National Task Force on the Prevention and Treatment of Obesity, "Weight Cycling," *JAMA* 272 (15, 19 Oct. 94):1196-1202.

10. Ardan Cockburn, *Mummies, Disease and Ancient Cultures*, Cambridge University Press (1980).

11. *US Bureau of the Census, Statistical Abstract* (Washington DC., 95):147, table 225.

12. Gina Kolata, "Benefit of Standard Low Fat Diet is Doubted," *New York Times*, (25 April 1995) 37.

13. U.S. Dept. of Agriculture, "What We Eat in America: 1994-96," (Feb., 96) 01.

14. Jacob C. Seidell, "Obesity in Europe: Scaling an Epidemic," *Intl. Journ. of Obesity,* 19 Supp. 3 (Sept. 95) 51-54.

15. Michael Fumento, *The Fat of the Land*, Penguin Books)1997) 64.

16. Joann Manson et al., "Body weight and Mortality Among Women," *NEJM* 333 (11, 14 Sept. 95):677-85.

17. Steven Whiting, *Self Health.*

18. Richard Heller, *The Carbohydrate Addict Gram Counter* (Signet Books 1993) v.

19. P.A.T. Southgate and J.V.G.A. Durnin, "Calorie Conversion Factors: An Experimental Reassessment of the Factors Used in the Calculation of the Energy Value of the Human Diet," *British Journal of Nutrition* 24 (1970) 517.

20. Dianne Partie Lange, *Allure Magazine* (Sept. 1999) 102.

21. Wayne C. Miller et al., "Dietary Fat, Sugar and Fiber Predict Body Fat Content," *Journal of the American Dietetic Assoc.* 94 (6, June 94):612-615.

22. James W. Anderson, "Dietary Fiber, Diabetes and Obesity," *American Journal of Gastroenterology* 81 (10, Oct. 86) 898-906.

23. Elizabeth Somer, *The Nutrition Desk Reference* (Keats Publishing 1995).

24. Debra Waterhouse, *Outsmarting the Female Fat Cell* (New York: Warner books 1993).

25. Fletcher, *Thin for Life*, (136).

26. Thomas A. Wadden et al., "Effects of Weight Cycling on the Resting Energy Expenditure and Body Composition of Obese Women," *Intl. Journal of Eating Disorders* 19 (1, Jan. 96) 5-12.

27. U.S. Senate, 74th Congress, Second session, Document No. 264.

28. Michael Colgan, *Your Personal Vitamin Profile* (1982).

29. 30. 31. 32. 33., As stated.

34. Losonczy, K.G. et al., "Vitamin E and Vitamin C Supplement Use and Risk of all Cause and Coronary Heart Disease and Mortality in Older Persons: the Established Populations for Epidemiologic Studies of the Elderly" *Am. Journal of /Clinical Nutrition* (1996; 64):190-6.

35. 36. 37., As stated.

38. Cooper, Kenneth, *Advanced Nutritional Therapies* (Thomas Nelson Publishers, 1996).

39. Cover of *Fortune Magazine* (July 1991)

40. *U.S. News and World Report*, Cover Story (9, Jan. 1995).

41. Eades, *Protein Power* (Bantam Books 1996) 300.

42. My assistant, Deborah Codute, in a phone conversation with Dr. De Fronzo during August 1999.

43. Scott Roberts, American Council on Exercise, *Personal Training Manual* (1996) 336.

44. Steven Whiting, "Osteoporosis," *Institute for Nutritional Science* (1997).

45. Jacqueline Berning, *Ace Book Sec Abu* 139.

46. Strause L. et al., "Spinal Bone Loss in Postmenopausal Women Supplemented with Calcium and Trace Minerals," *J. Nutri.* (1994) 124.

47. Steven Whiting, "How to Naturally Control Diabetes & Hypoglycemia," *Inst. for Nutr. Science* (1998).

48. A medical handout provided to doctors for their patients from the Eli Lilly Corp.

49. Mayo Clinic web sight information on diabetes.

50. Richard A. Anderson et al., "Elevated Intakes of Supplemental Chromium Improve Glucose and Insulin Variables In Individuals with Type II Diabetes," *Diabetes* (1997:46): 1786-1791.

51. 52. As stated.

52. Jason Theodosakis, *The Arthritis Cure*, (St. Martins Press, 1997).

Curves®

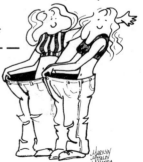